Your bloodstream is designed to carry just one teaspoon of sugar at any time. Most people consume thirty or forty teaspoons a day. The excess triggers a hormone called insulin. When insulin stays elevated for years, it quietly drives cancer, Alzheimer's, heart disease, diabetes, and more. Almost nobody tests for it. Almost everything about it is reversible. That is what this book is about.

THE INSULIN PROBLEM

Disclaimer

This book is not a substitute for medical advice. If you have any health concerns, or if you are on prescribed medication, please speak to your doctor before making changes based on what you read here. If the guidance in this book differs significantly from your current lifestyle, discuss it with your GP to determine whether it is right for you.

The author accepts no responsibility for any medical or health consequences that may arise from following the information in this book.

What works for one person may not work for another. Nothing in these pages is intended to override your doctor's advice or replace prescribed medication. If you are considering changes to your medication, seek opinions from more than one medical professional.

You are encouraged to share the insights from this book with your doctor and hear their perspective on its relevance to your health.

First published in Great Britain in 2026 by Clubwell

***Cover quote.** *Burden of Diseases, Injuries, and Risk Factors Among US States doi: 10.1001/jama.2018.0158*

Also by Steve Bennett

Primal Cure

Britain is Sick

Fat & Furious

Primal Gourmet

MARS

The Fibre First Diet

Sugar Tolerance

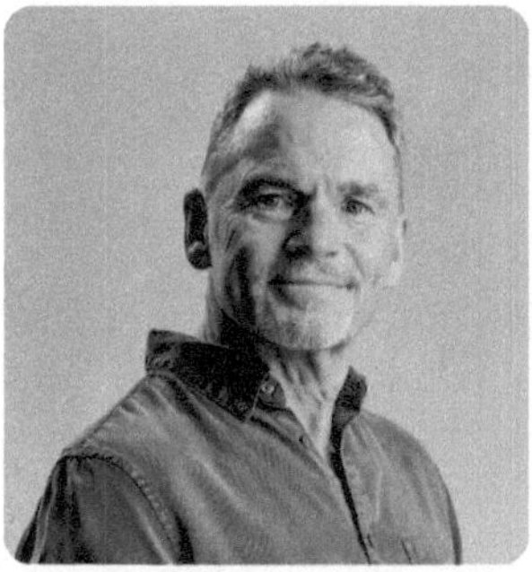

Steve Bennett is a British entrepreneur who has featured on the Sunday Times Fast Track 100 twice, topping the list in 2012. He has run four marathons fasted, sailed the Atlantic, walked to the North Pole, and spent the last decade researching metabolic health alongside leading scientists.

Now he is taking on his biggest challenge yet: proving that you cannot out-medicate chronic diseases. The answer was never pharmaceutical drugs. It is a single hormone.

And almost nobody is testing for it.

Dedicated to the researchers, scientists, and truth-seekers whose work made this book possible. I carry a responsibility to share what you have discovered and taught me as widely as possible.

ISBN 978-1-918852-00-4 (paperback)
ISBN 978-1-918852-01-1 (hardback)
ISBN 978-1-918852-02-8 (ebook)
ISBN 978-1-918852-03-5 (audiobook)

THE INSULIN PROBLEM

32 Diseases. One Cause.

STEVE BENNETT

Clubwell

Contents

Introduction

. . .

On the morning of 29 February 2024, as I made my way to the office, my phone started behaving like a popcorn machine on overdrive, bursting with alerts non-stop. Sensing something significant, I pulled over into a lay-by. Messages were flooding in from my doctor friends, with phrases like "We are winning," "Our voices are finally getting heard," "Down with UPFs," "They should have published your afflictions tree," and "You need to include this in your new book."

I had no idea what they were all talking about until I found a link to The Telegraph newspaper. There it was, in stark black and white: "Ultra-processed foods linked to more than 30 illnesses."

It was not just The Telegraph, either. The Daily Mail ran with "Ultra-processed foods are harmful to EVERY part of the body." The Guardian headlined "Ultra-processed food linked to 32 harmful effects to health." Even The Sun weighed in: "Full list of 32 health dangers lurking in your favourite foods."

So, what was behind all this buzz? The day before, the BMJ (British Medical Journal) had published one of the most significant nutritional studies to date. Ten million participants. A review so large and so thorough that it could no longer be dismissed as fringe science or cherry-picked data. The conclusion was devastating in its simplicity: modern foods are connected to 32 separate health conditions, from cancer and heart disease to anxiety and early death.

For me, that morning was bittersweet. On one hand, I felt vindicated. I had spent years researching, writing, and frankly shouting from the rooftops that our modern food supply was making us sick. My *Tree of Afflictions*, which mapped how insulin resistance branches out into dozens of chronic diseases, had been called alarmist by some. Well, here was the BMJ saying exactly the same thing with ten million people behind it.

On the other hand, I felt frustrated. Because knowing that food choices cause 32 diseases is only half the story. The question nobody in those headlines was answering was: why? What is the biological mechanism that connects a packet of biscuits to cancer, to diabetes, to depression, to liver disease? How does one dietary choice ripple out into so many different conditions?

That is what this book sets out to answer. But before we get there, I need to clear something up.

While it is good news that people are finally waking up to the fact that food is at the heart of these diseases, simply blaming ultra-processed food is a little wide of the mark. Not all UPF is the enemy. Bone broth would technically be classified as ultra-processed because of the process it goes through, yet it is one of the healthiest things you can consume. The real issue is not the level of processing. It is what that processing does to your insulin. Yes, many ultra-processed foods are stuffed with chemicals that are harmful in their own right. But the label alone does not tell you what you need to know.

And it is certainly not about calories. The government is obsessed with calorie counting, and I can tell you from conversations on the inside that this obsession is only going to get worse in the years ahead. But calories have very little to do with it. You could increase your calories from healthy foods that do not spike your insulin, and you would not drive any of these 32 diseases. Meanwhile, you could slash your calories dramatically, but if what you eat keeps insulin elevated, you are potentially heading for every single one of them.

The other obsession is what the government calls HFSS: foods high in fat, sugar, and salt. Their latest obesity strategy document is built around it. Just like the traffic light labelling system we already have on food packaging, this is wide of the mark. As you will read in these pages, excessive salt is potentially not the villain it has been made out to be. And high-quality fat is not a problem at all. The only part of that equation that holds up is excessive sugar. One out of three is not a great batting average for a national health strategy.

So yes, it is progress that food is finally being recognised as the cause of these diseases. But frustratingly, the conversation is still missing the main point. It is not about ultra-processing. It is not about calories. It is not about fat or salt. It is the insulin.

If I were writing this book a hundred years ago, it would have been about infectious diseases. Pneumonia, tuberculosis, polio, typhoid, diarrhoea. These were the killers. You either survived them or you did not. There would be no chapter on cancer. No chapter on heart disease, diabetes, dementia, or obesity. None of the conditions we discuss in this book would have concerned you, because they barely existed. Something has changed.

Medical science conquered the acute infections that once cut lives short, and we should be grateful for that. But in their place, an entirely new category of illness has emerged. Slow, creeping, chronic diseases that do not strike suddenly but build quietly over decades. And unlike the infections of the past, you cannot fix them with a pharmaceutical approach. There is no course of antibiotics for obesity, no vaccine for type 2 diabetes, no pill that reverses heart disease. These are lifestyle diseases, and they demand a lifestyle solution. That is what the following pages are all about.

This book is a follow-on to my earlier work, *The Fibre First Diet* and *Sugar Tolerance*. If you have read either of these, consider this the deeper dive into the science that underpins everything in those pages. If you have not, do not worry. You will still be able to follow along perfectly well.

Over the following chapters, you are going to meet Dr Isabella Cooper and Professor Ben Bikman, two brilliant scientists who helped me piece together the full picture. With what I have learnt through their metabolic research, I will walk you through the biological pathways that connect what you eat to how your body breaks down.

I have done my best to explain things in plain English throughout, and the glossary at the front is there for any terms that trip you up. Fair warning though: there are moments where we go properly into the biology. Mitochondria, insulin signalling, hormonal pathways. It gets a little sciency in places. But stick with it, because once you see how these pieces connect, you will never look at food the same way again.

I should warn you that in places this book pulls no punches. I have not softened the science to make it more comfortable, and I have not tiptoed around the failures of the institutions that should be protecting your health. Some of what you read will make you angry. It should. Too many books and too many experts have tried so hard to be diplomatic that the message gets watered down to the point where nobody acts on it. I would rather be blunt and save a life than be polite and lose one. If that means upsetting a few people along the way, I can live with that.

I should also say this. Science moves. It always has. In health, theories evolve, new enzymes and hormones are discovered, and biological pathways get refined or redrawn. It is possible that some of the specific mechanisms described in this book will be updated as research advances. That is how good science works. But the fundamentals will not change. Chronically elevated insulin drives chronic disease. Reducing it through what you eat and how you live reverses the damage. That is not a hypothesis waiting to be overturned. It is supported by decades of clinical evidence, thousands of published studies, and the personal experience of millions of people who have transformed their health by making this single change.

Whatever the science adds or adjusts in the years ahead, the core message of this book will hold.

And a note on references. My previous book, *The Fibre First Diet*, contained over 500 citations. This book takes a different approach. I have deliberately written it as a conversation, not a textbook, and I did not want footnotes and reference numbers breaking the flow every few sentences. Instead, wherever appropriate, I have named the researchers, the studies, and the institutions as I go. If I mention a study, I tell you who conducted it and when. If I quote a scientist, I tell you their name and credentials. In places where I have drawn on broader scientific consensus rather than a single source, I have not always named every reference individually, but the underlying research is well established and widely available. The Clubwell website hosts links to a vast array of research papers supporting the science in this book, and we are adding to it all the time.

I should be clear about something before we go any further. I am not claiming that insulin resistance directly causes all 32 of those diseases. Making that claim would be dishonest, and the science is more nuanced than that.

Some of these conditions are directly caused by insulin resistance. Type 2 diabetes is the most obvious. It is insulin resistance. Fatty liver disease is another, the direct result of the liver converting excess sugar into fat. Obesity, metabolic syndrome, PCOS, all have insulin resistance as a primary driver.

Others have multiple causes, but insulin resistance is almost always present and almost always making things worse.

Alzheimer's is a good example. There are genetic factors, lifestyle factors, and other contributors. But the research increasingly shows that insulin resistance in the brain plays a significant role, which is why some researchers now call it type 3 diabetes. The same is true for many cancers. Cancer has many triggers. But as you will read in Chapter 4, chronically high insulin drives cell growth and switches off the body's ability to destroy damaged cells. It does not necessarily start the fire, but it pours petrol on it.

Then there are conditions where insulin resistance may not be the primary cause but is so consistently present alongside them that it is difficult to call it a coincidence. Heart disease, stroke, chronic kidney disease, depression, anxiety. Look at the data and you will find insulin resistance sitting in the background of almost every case.

So here is the honest answer. Insulin resistance directly causes some of these diseases, significantly worsens most of the others, and is present in nearly all of them. Whether it lit the match or simply fanned the flames, it is involved. And the good news is that it is the one factor you can do something about, starting with your next meal.

By the end of this book, you will understand why those 32 diseases share one answer. And more importantly, you will know what to do about it.

Reference Section

. . .

This book is full of science. That is deliberate. I believe you deserve to understand what is happening inside your own body, not just be told what to eat. But science comes with its own vocabulary, and it feels like the medical profession has spent centuries making sure nobody outside the room can follow the conversation.

Some of the terms in the chapters ahead might be unfamiliar. That is why I have put this reference section at the front of the book rather than buried at the back where nobody ever looks. To help you along the way, whenever I first use a technical term, or reintroduce one after a while, I will put it in *italics* as a gentle nudge that it is explained here. You do not need to memorise any of this. Think of it as a reference you can come back to whenever a term trips you up. I have written it the way I would explain these things over a cup of coffee, not the way a textbook would.

If you are anything like me, you will want to dive straight in, so just skip ahead to Chapter 1 on page 41.

. . .

Aldosterone A hormone produced by your adrenal glands that tells your kidneys to retain sodium and water. It is part of your body's blood pressure regulation system. The problem is that chronically high insulin stimulates aldosterone production, causing your kidneys to hold onto more fluid than they should. This raises blood pressure. It is one of the reasons so many people with insulin resistance end up on blood pressure medication, treating the symptom while the insulin that is driving it goes unaddressed.

ALT (alanine aminotransferase) A liver enzyme that your doctor measures on a standard blood test. When liver cells are damaged or inflamed, they leak ALT into the bloodstream, so a raised level is a sign your liver is under stress. The problem is the reference ranges. In the UK, anything up to 30 for women and 50 for men is considered normal. But as you will discover in this book, in Dr Isabella Cooper's KetoSAge study, genuinely healthy participants had levels below 14. Your doctor could look at a result of 25, tell you everything is fine, and miss early fatty liver disease entirely.

AMPK (AMP-activated protein kinase) Your body's fuel gauge. When energy is low, during exercise, fasting, or when your cells need more power, AMPK switches on and tells your body to burn fat, absorb glucose, repair damaged cells, and build new mitochondria. When insulin is chronically high, AMPK stays suppressed. Many of the benefits described in this book, from autophagy to improved insulin sensitivity after exercise, are driven by AMPK activation.

Amyloid plaques Sticky protein clumps that accumulate in the brains of Alzheimer's patients. They are widely blamed for the disease, but decades of drugs targeting amyloid have failed. Growing evidence suggests that insulin resistance in the brain may be what triggers the buildup in the first place.

Angiogenesis The growth of new blood vessels. Cancer tumours hijack this process to build their own blood supply. Insulin and IGF-1 stimulate it, which is one of the pathways linking insulin resistance to cancer growth.

Apoptosis Programmed cell death. Healthy cells are designed to die when they are damaged or no longer needed. Cancer cells disable this self-destruct mechanism, allowing them to survive and multiply. Insulin resistance disrupts the process.

Aromatase An enzyme that converts testosterone into oestrogen. It is found in fat tissue, which means the more body fat you carry, the more aromatase you produce, and the more oestrogen you make. This is one of the reasons obesity is linked to hormone-driven cancers, particularly breast cancer in post-menopausal women. Insulin makes it worse. High insulin drives fat storage, more fat produces more aromatase, more aromatase produces more oestrogen, and excess oestrogen stimulates cell growth in breast and uterine tissue. It is a vicious circle that starts, once again, with insulin.

AST (aspartate aminotransferase) A liver enzyme measured alongside ALT. AST is found in the liver but also in the heart, muscles, and kidneys, so a raised level does not always point to the liver alone. When both AST and ALT are elevated together, it is a stronger signal that the liver is in trouble. The same problem with reference ranges applies. What your doctor calls normal may already be a sign that fat is building up in your liver and insulin resistance is taking hold.

Atherosclerosis The buildup of plaque inside your artery walls. Contrary to popular belief, it is not caused by eating fat. It is driven by chronic inflammation and insulin resistance damaging the artery lining.

ATP (adenosine triphosphate - from tri = three, phosphate = energy-carrying molecule) The energy currency of every cell in your body. Everything your cells do, contracting a muscle, firing a nerve, building a protein, requires ATP. Your mitochondria produce it by burning glucose, fatty acids, or ketones through the Krebs cycle and oxidative phosphorylation. A healthy cell extracts around 36 ATP molecules from a single molecule of glucose using this process. By contrast, glycolysis alone, without the mitochondria finishing the job, produces just 2. That is the difference between your cells running on a full engine and running on fumes.

Autophagy Your body's cellular recycling programme. It clears out damaged cells and components, making way for new ones. It is triggered by fasting and low insulin states and suppressed by constant eating and high insulin.

BAX (BCL-2 Associated X protein) A death protein and the opposite of BCL-2. When a cell is damaged, BAX punches holes in the mitochondrial membrane, triggering apoptosis, the cell's self-destruct sequence. In a healthy body, BAX ensures that broken cells are eliminated before they cause harm. When insulin is chronically high, BAX is suppressed while BCL-2 is amplified, meaning damaged cells survive when they should not. It is one of the ways insulin resistance disables your body's natural defence against cancer.

BCL-2 (B-cell lymphoma 2) A survival protein inside every cell whose job is to keep the cell alive. It sits in a constant tug of war with its opposite, BAX. In a healthy body, BCL-2 protects cells that are still useful and steps aside when they are damaged beyond repair. The problem is that chronically high insulin upregulates BCL-2, tipping the balance in favour of survival. Cells that should be destroyed are kept alive instead, including cells with damaged DNA that could become cancerous.

Blood-brain barrier (BBB) A tightly sealed wall of cells that protects your brain by controlling what gets in and what stays out. Nutrients like DHA need specific transport vehicles to cross it, so too does insulin. Chronic insulin resistance damages this barrier, allowing toxins and inflammatory molecules through and contributing to Alzheimer's and other neurodegenerative diseases.

Cholesterol A waxy, fat-like substance that your body makes in large quantities because it needs it. Every cell membrane in your body contains cholesterol. Your brain is roughly 25% cholesterol by dry weight. It is the raw material for vitamin D, testosterone, oestrogen, cortisol, and bile acids. Without it, you would die. Your liver manufactures around 80% of the cholesterol in your body regardless of what you eat, and when you eat more, your liver simply makes less. The idea that dietary cholesterol clogs your arteries has been quietly abandoned by most serious researchers, though the message has not reached the public. Cholesterol is transported through your blood in particles called lipoproteins: VLDL, LDL, and HDL. It is the type and size of these particles, not the total cholesterol number, that matters. As you will read in Chapter 6, the real driver of heart disease is not cholesterol. It is insulin, inflammation, and the damage they do to your arterial walls.

Cortisol Your stress hormone. Short bursts are useful: they sharpen focus and release energy. But chronic stress keeps cortisol elevated, which drives up blood sugar and insulin. It is one of the reasons stress makes you gain weight around the middle, even if your diet has not changed.

CRP (C-reactive protein) A protein produced by your liver that rises sharply when there is inflammation anywhere in your body. Doctors use it as a general marker of inflammation, and it is one of the few inflammatory markers routinely tested on a standard blood panel. The problem is that most doctors treat elevated CRP as a standalone finding, prescribing anti-inflammatories without asking what is driving the inflammation in the first place. In the context of this book, the answer is almost always the same: chronically elevated insulin. Insulin drives chronic low-grade inflammation, which drives CRP up, which accelerates damage to your arteries, your joints, your brain, and just about every other tissue in your body. If your CRP is elevated, do not just treat the inflammation. Ask why it is there.

De novo lipogenesis (de novo = from new, lipo = fat, genesis = creation) The process by which your liver converts excess sugar, particularly fructose, directly into fat. Most people assume fruit juice is healthy, but a glass of orange juice delivers a concentrated fructose hit that your liver processes in much the same way it processes alcohol.

DHA (docosahexaenoic acid) An omega-3 fatty acid that makes up a large proportion of your brain's structure. Your body cannot make enough of it on its own, so it must come from your diet, primarily oily fish, shellfish, or high-quality supplements.

DNA (deoxyribonucleic acid) The instruction manual inside every cell in your body. It contains the complete blueprint for building and running you. Every time a cell divides, it has to copy the entire manual. Normally your body is meticulous about this, checking for errors and repairing damage before allowing the copy to go ahead. But when insulin is chronically high and *m*TOR is stuck in the on position, cells divide too fast for the quality checks to keep up. Errors creep in. If enough errors accumulate in the wrong places, a normal cell can become a cancerous one. That is why the repair window, the quiet period when *m*TOR is turned down, matters so much. As you will read in Chapter 4, DNA damage may not be the cause of cancer, but rather a consequence of something deeper: broken mitochondria.

Eatwell Guide The UK government's official dietary guidelines, still in use despite being hopelessly outdated. It recommends that roughly 50% of your diet should come from carbohydrates, mainly bread, rice, pasta, and potatoes. You could just as easily call it the SUK Diet, the Standard UK Diet, because that is exactly what most people follow. As you will read in this book, that recommendation is one of the main drivers of virtually every chronic disease we discuss.

Enzymes Proteins that make chemical reactions happen in your body. They speed up processes that would otherwise be too slow to sustain life. Every process in this book involves enzymes. Hormone-sensitive lipase is an enzyme that breaks down stored fat. Lipoprotein lipase is an enzyme that pulls fat from your blood into your cells. The enzymes in your mitochondria drive the Krebs cycle and produce ATP. Your liver uses enzymes to convert fructose into fat. Think of enzymes as the workers in a factory: the raw materials might be there, but nothing gets built without them.

Fibre The indigestible part of plant foods. It is not a nutrient in the traditional sense because your body cannot absorb it. Instead, it slows sugar absorption, feeds your gut bacteria, and stimulates GLP-1 production. It is nature's antidote to sugar.

Fructose The sugar found naturally in fruit but added in enormous quantities to processed food and drinks. Unlike glucose, fructose is processed almost entirely by your liver. In excess, it overwhelms the liver and is converted directly into fat through de novo lipogenesis. It is one of the primary drivers of fatty liver disease.

GLP-1 (glucagon-like peptide-1) A hormone your gut produces naturally when you eat real food. It tells your brain you are full and slows digestion so you stay satisfied. The weight loss injections are synthetic versions of this hormone, dialled up to unnatural levels.

Glucagon Insulin's opposite. When blood sugar drops, your pancreas releases glucagon, which tells the liver to release stored glucose back into the bloodstream. Think of them as a seesaw: when insulin is up, glucagon is down, and your body stores energy. When insulin drops, glucagon rises, and your body releases it. The problem with chronic hyperinsulinaemia is that insulin never drops low enough for glucagon to do its job properly.

Glucomannan A viscous fibre that expands to fifty times its weight in water. It is the only fibre with approved weight loss claims from the European Food Safety Authority. It physically stretches the gut wall, triggers L-cells, and slows carbohydrate absorption.

Gluconeogenesis (gluco = glucose, neo = new, genesis = creation) The process by which your liver creates brand new glucose from non-sugar sources, primarily amino acids from protein. This is how your body maintains blood sugar even when you eat no carbohydrates at all. It is a normal and essential process. The problem arises when the liver becomes insulin resistant and gluconeogenesis runs unchecked, pumping glucose into your bloodstream around the clock, even when blood sugar is already high. This is one of the main reasons fasting blood sugar creeps up in people with insulin resistance.

Glucose (from the Greek glukus = sweet) The simplest form of sugar and the most basic energy molecule in nature. Plants make it from sunlight through photosynthesis, and virtually every living thing on earth uses it for fuel. A single molecule of glucose is extraordinarily small, far too small to see, yet it is the molecule your body monitors more tightly than almost anything else. Here is the important part: you do not have to eat it. Your body can manufacture all the glucose it needs from protein through a process called gluconeogenesis. Your liver does this around the clock. So when someone tells you that you need carbohydrates for energy, the correct response is: no, you do not. Your body has been making its own glucose since the day you were born.

GLUT1 A glucose transporter that is always open, regardless of insulin. It is found on cells that need a constant fuel supply, like red blood cells and brain cells. Cancer cells upregulate GLUT1 to feed their appetite for sugar, which is why they can keep growing even when insulin signalling is disrupted elsewhere.

GLUT4 A glucose transporter that acts as a door on muscle and fat cells. It only opens when insulin tells it to. In insulin resistance, these doors become stiff and unresponsive, so glucose builds up in the bloodstream instead. This is the transporter that locks shut when your cells stop listening to insulin.

Glycation What happens when excess sugar in your blood sticks to proteins and fats, creating damaged molecules called AGEs (advanced glycation end-products). It is like sugar caramelising inside your body, stiffening blood vessels and accelerating ageing.

Glycerol-3-phosphate (glycerol = the backbone of fat, phosphate = energy-carrying molecule) The scaffolding that holds fat molecules together. Think of it as the frame of a parcel. Fatty acids are the contents, but without glycerol-3-phosphate to bind them into a triglyceride, they cannot be packaged and stored. Your body makes glycerol-3-phosphate from glucose, which is why eating carbohydrates does not just raise your blood sugar, it also gives your fat cells the very material they need to lock fat away.

Glycogen The body's short-term energy store, made from chains of glucose molecules packed tightly together. Your liver holds around 100 grams and your muscles around 400 grams. When blood sugar drops, your liver breaks glycogen back into glucose and releases it into your bloodstream. Once these stores are full, any excess glucose is converted to fat through *de novo lipogenesis*. Think of glycogen as your quick-access current account and body fat as your long-term savings account.

Glycogenolysis (glycogen = stored glucose, lysis = breaking apart) The breaking down of glycogen, your body's short-term glucose store, back into glucose for release into the bloodstream. Your liver holds roughly 100 grams of glycogen, enough to keep your brain and red blood cells fuelled for about 24 hours. In a healthy body, insulin tells the liver when to stop breaking down glycogen. In an insulin-resistant liver, that signal is ignored, and glycogenolysis continues even when it should not, adding yet more glucose to a bloodstream that already has too much.

HbA1c (glycated haemoglobin) (haemo = blood, globin = protein) A blood test that measures how much sugar has stuck to your red blood cells over the previous two to three months. Because red blood cells live for about 120 days, HbA1c gives your doctor a rolling average of your blood sugar rather than a single snapshot. It is the test most commonly used to diagnose and monitor type 2 diabetes. The problem is that HbA1c only measures glucose. It tells you nothing about insulin. A person can have a perfectly normal HbA1c while their insulin levels are through the roof, because the pancreas is still managing to force blood sugar down. By the time HbA1c starts to rise, insulin resistance has often been doing its damage silently for years, sometimes decades.

HDL (high-density lipoprotein) Often called "good cholesterol," though it is not actually cholesterol. It is a transport particle. HDL's job is to collect excess cholesterol from your tissues and carry it back to the liver for recycling or disposal. Think of it as the cleanup crew. Higher HDL is generally associated with better cardiovascular health, and one of the most reliable ways to raise it is to reduce carbohydrates and increase healthy fats. A ketogenic diet almost always pushes HDL up.

HIF-1α (hypoxia-inducible factor 1 alpha) (hypoxia = low oxygen, inducible = can be switched on) A protein that acts as an emergency switch when a cell detects low oxygen levels. In a healthy body, HIF-1α triggers the growth of new blood vessels to restore oxygen supply. Cancer cells hijack this system. Because they ferment glucose instead of using oxygen, they behave as though they are suffocating, even when oxygen is plentiful. This triggers HIF-1α, which tells the body to build new blood vessels directly to the tumour, feeding it with the glucose and nutrients it needs to grow. Insulin and IGF-1 both upregulate HIF-1α, which is yet another way chronically high insulin helps cancer build its own supply lines.

Hormone-sensitive lipase (HSL) An enzyme that works inside your fat cells. Its job is to break down stored triglycerides into free fatty acids so they can be released back into the bloodstream and burned for fuel. When insulin is low,

HSL switches on and your fat stores open up. When insulin is high, HSL is suppressed and your stored fat is locked in.

Hyper vs Hypo (hyper = too much, hypo = too little) Two prefixes the medical world uses constantly, and they are easy to confuse. Hyper means excess. Hypo means not enough. So, hyperinsulinaemia means too much insulin in the blood. Hypoinsulinaemia means too little. Hyperglycaemia means blood sugar is too high. Hypoglycaemia means it has dropped too low. Hyperthyroidism means an overactive thyroid. Hypothyroidism means an underactive one. Once you know these two prefixes, half the medical vocabulary in this book unlocks itself.

Hyperinsulinaemia Chronically elevated insulin levels in the blood. This is the state that drives fat storage, inflammation, and the cascade of diseases described in this book. Your doctor may not test for it directly, which is part of the problem.

IGF-1 (insulin-like growth factor 1) A growth hormone triggered by insulin. When insulin is chronically high, IGF-1 stays elevated too, sending a constant grow and divide signal to your cells. This is one of the key pathways linking insulin resistance to cancer. Healthy cells respond to it normally. Cancer cells exploit it.

Inflammation (chronic) A low-grade, persistent immune response that damages your own tissues over time. Acute inflammation heals a cut or fights an infection. Chronic inflammation, driven by sugar, seed oils, and insulin resistance, is a root cause of virtually every modern disease.

Insulin A hormone made by your pancreas. Its main job is to clear sugar out of your blood and store it. When insulin is chronically high, your body gets locked in fat storage mode and cannot burn its own reserves. It is the central villain of this book.

Insulin resistance What happens when your cells stop responding properly to insulin. Your pancreas has to produce more and more of it to get the same result. Over time, this leads to chronically elevated insulin levels, which drive the cascade of damage described in this book. This is the trunk of the tree.

Ketogenic diet A way of eating that keeps carbohydrates very low, forcing the body to burn fat for fuel and enter ketosis. Isabella's KetoSAge study demonstrates how a keto diet improves virtually every metabolic marker of health.

Ketones An alternative fuel your body produces when insulin is low and carbohydrate intake is restricted. Your liver makes ketones by breaking down fatty acids released from your fat stores. Your brain, heart, and muscles can all run on ketones efficiently. Measuring ketones in your blood, breath, or urine is a reliable indicator that your insulin levels are low enough for your body to be accessing its own fat reserves. This state is called ketosis.

KetoSAge Dr Isabella Cooper's landmark study that tested what happens when healthy people in ketosis switch to the government's recommended high-carbohydrate diet. The results were dramatic and form the scientific backbone of this book.

Ketosis A metabolic state where your body burns fat for fuel instead of sugar, producing molecules called ketones. It is proof that your insulin is low. You can measure it with a simple breath, blood, or urine test.

Krebs cycle (also called the citric acid cycle) The engine room inside your mitochondria where fuel is converted into energy. Once glucose, fatty acids, ketones, or amino acids have been broken down into a molecule called acetyl-CoA, the Krebs cycle takes over, spinning that molecule through a series of chemical reactions that strip out electrons. Those electrons are then passed to the next stage, oxidative phosphorylation, where the real energy production happens. It is a beautifully efficient system when it is working properly.

L-cells Specialised cells lining your small intestine that produce GLP-1 when stimulated by food, particularly fibre and protein. They are your body's natural version of what the pharmaceutical industry is now selling for billions. The difference is that your L-cells produce GLP-1 in small, measured amounts at exactly the right time.

LDL (low-density lipoprotein) Often called "bad cholesterol," though the story is far more complicated than you have been told. LDL is the shrunken remains of a VLDL particle after it has delivered its fat cargo. Not all LDL is the same. Large, buoyant LDL particles are generally harmless. Small, dense LDL particles are the ones associated with heart disease because they can burrow into damaged arterial walls and trigger inflammation. What drives the production of small dense LDL? High insulin, high triglycerides, and a diet full of sugar and refined carbohydrates. Not saturated fat. The standard cholesterol tests your doctor runs do not distinguish between the two types, which is one of the reasons the cholesterol story has been so badly misunderstood for so long.

Leptin A hormone produced by your fat cells that tells your brain you have enough energy stored and can stop eating. In theory, the more fat you carry, the louder the signal. In practice, chronic insulin resistance causes leptin resistance too, so your brain never gets the message. You stay hungry even when your body has more than enough fuel.

Lipase A general term for any enzyme that breaks down fat. Your body has several, each with a different job. Pancreatic lipase breaks down the fat you eat. Lipoprotein lipase (LPL) sits on the surface of your cells and pulls fat from the bloodstream. Hormone-sensitive lipase (HSL) works inside your fat cells, releasing stored fat to be burned. The two that matter most in this book are HSL and LPL, because insulin controls both of them, in opposite directions.

Lipoprotein lipase (LPL) An enzyme that sits on the outer surface of your fat cells. Its job is to grab triglycerides from the bloodstream and pull the fatty acids inside for storage. When insulin is high, LPL is highly active and your fat cells are pulling in fat from every direction. When insulin is low, LPL quiets down and the entrance to your fat cells slows.

MAPK pathway (mitogen-activated protein kinase) One of two signalling routes activated when insulin binds to its receptor, the other being the PI3K pathway. MAPK controls cell growth and division. When insulin is chronically elevated, the MAPK pathway is constantly switched on, telling cells to grow and multiply. It is one of the mechanisms by which insulin resistance drives tumour development.

Melatonin Best known as the sleep hormone, produced by the tiny pineal gland in the centre of your brain when darkness falls. But it is also one of the most powerful antioxidants your body produces. It protects your mitochondria overnight. Blue light from screens suppresses it, which is why evening screen time damages more than just your sleep.

Metabolic rate (also basal metabolic rate, BMR) The speed at which your body burns energy at rest. Your basal metabolic rate is the baseline, the energy your body uses just to keep you alive: breathing, pumping blood, maintaining body temperature. When you lose weight by simply eating less, your metabolic rate can drop and stay low, making regain almost inevitable. Losing weight by reducing carbohydrates rather than just cutting calories appears to protect it.

Metabolic syndrome A cluster of conditions that occur together: high blood pressure, high blood sugar, excess body fat around the waist, and abnormal cholesterol levels. It dramatically increases your risk of heart disease, stroke, and type 2 diabetes. Metabolic syndrome and insulin resistance are so closely linked that many researchers consider them virtually inseparable. Where you find one, you almost always find the other. According to the latest data, 93% of American adults have at least one of the five markers of metabolic dysfunction. In the UK, I guess we are not far behind.

Methylation A chemical process where your body attaches a small molecule called a methyl group to your DNA, proteins, or other molecules. Think of it as a series of tiny on/off switches. When a methyl group is added to a gene, it can silence it. When it is removed, the gene becomes active again. This is how your body controls which genes are expressed and which stay quiet, without changing the DNA itself. It matters for this book because methylation is one of the ways your body keeps dangerous genes, including cancer-promoting genes, switched off. When methylation goes wrong, genes that should be silenced get switched back on. Insulin resistance, poor diet, stress, and toxin exposure can all disrupt methylation, which is one more way the modern lifestyle creates conditions that favour disease.

Microbiome The trillions of bacteria living in your gut. Roughly 80% of your immune system operates from here. Feed them fibre and they thrive. Feed them sugar and ultra-processed food and the balance shifts towards disease.

Mitochondria Tiny power stations inside almost every cell in your body. They convert food into energy. When they are damaged by chronic sugar overload or seed oils, you feel tired, your organs struggle, and disease follows.

***m*TOR (mechanistic target of rapamycin)** A master growth switch inside your cells. When *m*TOR is active, your cells are in building mode: growing, dividing, storing. When it is quiet, your body shifts into repair and recycling mode (autophagy). Chronic high insulin keeps *m*TOR permanently switched on, which accelerates ageing and creates conditions that favour cancer.

NAFLD / MAFLD (fatty liver disease) Fat accumulating in the liver, driven by excess sugar and carbohydrates. It now affects roughly one in three adults in the UK, and in children the numbers are rising fast. The condition was originally called non-alcoholic fatty liver disease (NAFLD), but in 2020 it was renamed MAFLD, metabolic dysfunction-associated fatty liver disease, because researchers finally acknowledged what drives it: not alcohol, but metabolic dysfunction. The new name alone tells you everything this book is about.

Omega-3 and omega-6 fatty acids Two families of essential fats your body needs but cannot make. Omega-3s (from fish, shellfish, and certain seeds) are anti-inflammatory. Omega-6s (concentrated in seed oils and processed food) are pro-inflammatory when consumed in excess. The modern diet contains roughly twenty times more omega-6 than omega-3, which drives chronic inflammation.

-opathy (from the Greek pathos = suffering or disease) A suffix the medical world attaches to almost everything to mean disease or damage. Once you know it, the words stop being intimidating. Retinopathy: disease of the retina (your eyes). Nephropathy: disease of the nephrons (your kidneys). Neuropathy: disease of the nerves. Cardiomyopathy: disease of the heart muscle. You will also see the word pathological in this book, which simply means caused by disease or related to disease. Every time you see a word ending in *opathy*, or the word pathological, just remember, pathos means suffering. The first half of the word tells you where.

Osteocalcin A hormone produced by your bones when you walk or do weight-bearing exercise. It helps regulate insulin sensitivity and plays a role in mood, energy, and metabolism. One of the reasons walking is so powerful.

PCOS (polycystic ovary syndrome) A hormonal condition affecting women's fertility and menstrual cycles. It is directly linked to insulin resistance. The ovaries' theca cells remain responsive to insulin even when other cells become resistant, leading to excess androgen production.

Pepsin A digestive enzyme produced by the lining of your stomach. Its sole job is to break down protein into smaller fragments called peptides. Pepsin only works in highly acidic conditions, which is why your stomach produces hydrochloric acid. When stomach acid is low, whether from ageing, stress, or long-term use of acid-suppressing drugs, pepsin cannot do its job properly and protein digestion suffers.

Peptides Short chains of amino acids created when digestive enzymes like pepsin break down the proteins you eat. Think of a protein as a long necklace and peptides as the smaller sections it gets snapped into. These shorter chains are then broken down further in the small intestine into individual amino acids, which your body absorbs and uses to build muscle, hormones, enzymes, and virtually every structure in your body.

PI3K (phosphoinositide 3-kinase) pathway One of two major signalling routes activated when insulin binds to a cell's receptor, the other being the MAPK pathway. PI3K handles the metabolic jobs: opening glucose transporters, storing energy, building proteins. When insulin is at normal levels, this pathway does exactly what it should. When insulin is chronically high, PI3K gets stuck in the on position, driving cell growth and keeping damaged cells alive when they should be dying. In cancer, this pathway is frequently mutated or overactivated, which is why pharmaceutical companies have spent billions trying to block it with drugs. Lowering insulin does it for free.

ROS (reactive oxygen species) Tiny, highly reactive molecules produced as a byproduct when your mitochondria generate energy. In small amounts they are useful, acting as signalling molecules and helping your immune system kill bacteria. But when production spirals out of control, ROS damage everything they touch: DNA, cell membranes, proteins, and the mitochondria themselves. This is what people mean when they talk about oxidative stress. Chronically high insulin drives excessive ROS production, which is one of the reasons insulin resistance accelerates ageing, damages blood vessels, and creates the kind of cellular chaos that cancer thrives in.

Seed oils Industrially processed vegetable oils such as soy, sunflower, rapeseed, and safflower oil. They are high in omega-6 fatty acids and drive chronic inflammation. They are in virtually every processed food product.

SHBG (sex hormone-binding globulin) A protein made by your liver that binds to testosterone and oestrogen, keeping them in check. When insulin is high, SHBG drops, leaving too much of these hormones unbound and active. In women, excess free testosterone drives PCOS, acne, and hair loss. In men, excess free oestrogen promotes fat storage, particularly around the chest and belly. Both trace back to the same cause: too much insulin suppressing the liver's production of SHBG.

Short-chain fatty acids (SCFAs) Molecules produced when gut bacteria ferment fibre. They nourish the cells lining your colon, regulate your immune system, and help control inflammation. Butyrate is the most important one.

Telomeres Protective caps on the ends of your chromosomes, like the plastic tips on shoelaces. They shorten every time a cell divides. Chronic inflammation and insulin resistance accelerate the shortening, effectively ageing you faster.

Tree of Afflictions My diagram showing how insulin resistance sits at the core of virtually every chronic disease. Its branches reach into cancer, heart disease, Alzheimer's, diabetes, fatty liver, gout, PCOS, and dozens more. Swiss Re, one of the world's largest reinsurance companies, endorsed it.

Triglycerides Fat molecules circulating in your blood. When you eat more sugar or refined carbohydrates than your body can burn, your liver converts the excess into triglycerides. High triglycerides are a direct signal that your liver is overwhelmed and your insulin is working overtime. One of the five key markers of metabolic health.

Type 2 diabetes The condition where your body can no longer control blood sugar effectively. It is not a disease you catch. It is the end stage of insulin resistance that has been building, often silently, for years or decades.

VLDL (very low-density lipoprotein — very low-density because it is large and full of fat, making it light for its size) A type of particle made by the liver to transport the fat it has just manufactured out into the bloodstream. When your liver converts excess glucose or fructose into fat through de novo lipogenesis, it packages that fat into VLDL particles and ships them out. The more sugar you eat, the more VLDL your liver produces. As VLDL travels through your bloodstream delivering its fat cargo, it shrinks. It becomes IDL (intermediate-density lipoprotein) and then shrinks further into LDL (low-density lipoprotein), the one your doctor measures on a cholesterol test. There is also HDL (high-density lipoprotein), which works in the opposite direction, collecting excess cholesterol from your tissues and carrying it back to the liver for disposal. The key insight for this book is that high VLDL and high triglycerides are not caused by eating fat. They are caused by eating too much sugar. Your standard cholesterol test will never tell you that.

Warburg effect The observation, first made by Otto Warburg in the 1920s, that cancer cells prefer to burn sugar for energy even when oxygen is available. Healthy cells use their mitochondria efficiently. Cancer cells rely on rapid, wasteful sugar burning instead, which is why they consume vastly more glucose than normal tissue. His observation, now called the Warburg effect, was largely ignored for decades but has experienced a major revival as the link between metabolism and cancer becomes undeniable.

CHAPTER ONE

The Tree Revisited

• • •

In my book *The Fibre First Diet*, I drew a picture of a tree. Not a pretty one. I'm no artist. But it became one of the most shared images from anything I've ever written.

The tree had a single trunk: insulin resistance. And from that trunk grew branches, each one a different disease. Heart disease on one branch. Type 2 diabetes on another. Alzheimer's. Cancer. Fatty liver disease. PCOS. Erectile dysfunction. High blood pressure. Gout. The list went on and on, spreading outward like a canopy of suffering, all growing from the same root.

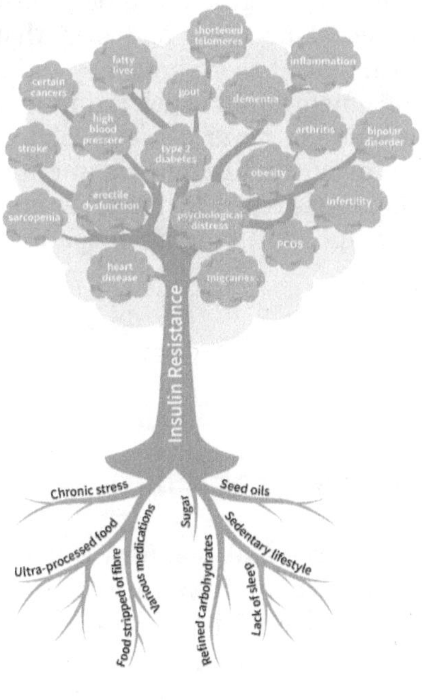

Swiss Re, the world's largest reinsurance company, endorsed that tree. Doctors at health conferences around the world started using it in their presentations. It was shown in the House of Lords here in the UK. And it was presented at the White House as part of the Make America Healthy Again movement. I'm certainly not claiming credit for what happened next, but just months after it was shown, America changed its food pyramid for the first time in decades. The seeds of my tree may have played a small part in that. Who knows.

The reason it resonates so powerfully is that it tells a simple truth that mainstream medicine has been slow to acknowledge: most of the chronic diseases destroying people's lives are not separate problems requiring separate drugs. They are different symptoms of the same underlying condition.

My good friend Professor Ben Bikman used almost identical language in an online podcast, which has been watched by millions of people. He described chronic diseases as "branches growing from the same tree" and said that conventional clinical care "will look at these branches and give someone a prescription for a medication which is only going to prune the branch back a little bit, never actually solving the problem." When I heard him say that I knew we were talking about the same thing. The tree is real. The branches are real. And until we stop pruning and start digging at the roots, nothing will change.

• • •

The Scale of the Problem

Professor Gerald Reaven at Stanford University spent sixty years researching insulin resistance. Sixty years. And his conclusion, published as far back as 1988, was clear:

Insulin resistance and compensatory hyperinsulinaemia play a central role in a cluster of metabolic abnormalities that underpin several of the most common chronic diseases of our time.

Those diseases? When you follow the science forward, the list expands: obesity. Arterial disease. Heart attack and stroke. Type 2 diabetes. High blood pressure. Fatty liver disease. Certain cancers. And dementia. Different conditions on the surface – but many share the same underlying metabolic dysfunction.

And here's the part that should make you sit up. Research has shown that insulin resistance multiplies the risk of Alzheimer's by five times. Cancer by up to twelve times. And death from cardiovascular disease by almost six times. Combined, if you have insulin resistance, the odds of developing at least one of these three conditions increase twenty-one-fold.

Let me say that again. Twenty-one times more likely. Not 21%. Twenty-one times.

And how many of us have insulin resistance? According to the latest data, 93% of American adults have at least one of the five markers associated with it. In the UK, I guess we are not far behind (no official data yet released). That means roughly nine out of every ten adults are walking around with this condition, and most of them are completely unaware.

• • •

The One Teaspoon Rule

To understand why insulin resistance has become so widespread, you need to understand one simple fact about your body. It is so important that I named an entire book after it.

Your entire bloodstream, all five litres of it running through sixty thousand miles of arteries and capillaries, is designed to carry just one teaspoon of sugar at any given time. That's it. Four to five grams. One teaspoon.

Everything beyond that single teaspoon is a problem. And insulin's primary job is to solve that problem. To get the excess sugar out of your blood before it causes damage. Because the damage is real and it is specific: excess glucose destroys the tiny blood vessels in your eyes (retinopathy), your kidneys (nephropathy), and the nerve endings in your feet and hands (neuropathy). It is why diabetes is the leading cause of blindness, kidney failure, and amputation in the developed world.

So, insulin pushes the excess sugar into your muscles and liver first. But those fill up fast. Once they are full, insulin converts the remaining sugar into body fat. That is not a design flaw. For most of human history, it was a survival mechanism. Our ancestors ate fruit in autumn, stored it as fat, and burned it through winter. Insulin was the hibernation hormone, and the system worked beautifully for two million years.

Then we invented supermarkets.

Today, a single bowl of cornflakes can dump the equivalent of eight to eighteen teaspoons of sugar (depends on the size of your bowl) into your bloodstream. Add a glass of apple juice and you can be consuming 24 teaspoons of sugar at the breakfast table. A jacket potato? Fifteen teaspoons. A foot-long Subway sandwich, just the bread? Another fifteen. And that is before lunch is over.

Let me be biologically clear here. I am saying that eating these foods and drinking these drinks has the same effect on your blood glucose level (glucose is the name for sugar in your blood) as eating that many teaspoons of sugar, straight out of a bag of table sugar.

The following three charts bring this to life. Most of the data is thanks to the great work of Dr David Unwin, and they show the effect on your blood sugar level when you eat these foods in these portions. Remember, your body is designed to carry just one teaspoon of sugar in your bloodstream at any given time.

The first chart shows a typical British breakfast. Real portions as per research we conducted for my previous book, not the tiny serving sizes on the box. Look at what a bowl of cornflakes, a glass of apple juice, and some milk does to your blood sugar before you have even left the house.

A healthy breakfast: cereal and fruit juice?

Breakfast	Serving	How does each food affect blood glucose compared with one 4g teaspoon of table sugar?
Cornflakes	69g	19
Milk added to Cornflakes	125ml	1
Sugar added to Cornflakes	1 tsp	1
Apple juice	200ml	8

Total blood sugar impact of breakfast: 29 teaspoons of sugar

And it is not just cornflakes. The second chart includes six popular breakfast cereals at the 30-gram serving size the manufacturers print on the packet. Even at that modest portion, most of them contain more sugar than a dessert. Now remember, nobody eats 30 grams. Most people pour two or three times that amount.

Breakfast	Serving	Table sugar teaspoon equivalent
Cornflakes	30g*	8.4
Coco Pops	30g*	7.3
Shredded Wheat	30g*	4.8
Bran Flakes	30g*	4.8
Mini Wheats	30g*	4.4
Oat Porridge	150g	4.4
Special K	30g*	4
Brown Toast	1 slice	3.3

The third chart moves to lunch and dinner. If you are looking for something to focus on, something that surprises most people I talk to, look at what a single jacket potato does to your blood sugar level.

Food item	Serving	Table sugar teaspoon equivalent
Jacket Potato	Large	15
12" Subway (just bread)	150g	15
Orange Juice	250ml	6
Basmati Rice	150g	10
Potato White (boiled)	150g	9.1
French Fries (baked)	150g	7.5
Spaghetti White (boiled)	180g	6.6
Sandwich (just the bread)	60g	7.4

Your body is calibrated for one teaspoon. And we are hammering it with twenty, thirty, sometimes forty teaspoons a meal, every day, year after year.

Now, if you are not sure what insulin actually is, here it is in plain English. Insulin is a hormone. It is made by your pancreas, a small organ tucked behind your stomach. And one of its main roles is straightforward: to regulate your blood sugar. When sugar enters your bloodstream after a meal, insulin is released to bring it back down to that safe one teaspoon level. It does this by signalling your cells to open their doors and let the sugar in, where it can be used for energy. Insulin does not physically carry the sugar. It is more like a key that unlocks the door. Without the key, the sugar stays in your bloodstream. With it, your cells open up and take what they need.

If there is still too much sugar for your cells to use, another of insulin's roles is to signal your liver to convert the excess into fat and store it. That is insulin doing its job. The problem is not insulin itself. The problem is that we are forcing it to work non-stop, meal after meal, snack after snack, day after day, with no rest. The insulin system never gets a break. It is being asked to do overtime every single day of your life.

• • •

From Resistance to Disease

When any system is overloaded for long enough, it starts to break. In biology, persistence nearly always leads to resistance. And insulin is no different. Imagine your body's cells as houses, and insulin as a postman knocking on the door to deliver sugar. At first, the doors open quickly. The sugar goes in. No problem. But when the postman is knocking constantly – morning, noon, night, with every snack, every sugary drink, every slice of white bread – eventually the cells stop answering the door. They've had enough. They're full.

That's insulin resistance. Your cells are no longer responding properly to insulin's signal. So, your pancreas does what any frustrated postmaster would do: it sends more postmen. More insulin. Louder knocking. And for a while, it works.

The extra insulin forces the sugar through. Your blood sugar tests come back normal. Your doctor tells you everything looks fine.

But everything is not fine. Because while your blood sugar may look normal, your insulin levels are through the roof. Your body is hiding the problem. The sugar is under control, yes, but only because insulin is working overtime to keep it there. And it is that excess insulin, the *hyperinsulinaemia*, that is now causing a completely different kind of damage. Not to the small blood vessels in your eyes, kidneys, and nerves – that is what high sugar does. High insulin attacks on a much broader front: driving fat storage, fuelling inflammation, triggering cell growth, and laying the groundwork for cancer, Alzheimer's, and heart disease. The irony is cruel. By the time your doctor finally spots the sugar problem, the insulin has been doing its damage silently for years.

This is the critical insight that mainstream medicine has been painfully slow to grasp. We have been measuring the wrong thing. For decades, doctors have tested blood sugar and *HbA1c* as the gold standard for metabolic health. But you can have perfectly normal blood sugar while your elevated insulin is silently destroying you from the inside. The sugar looks fine because the insulin is working overtime to keep it down. It's like checking the water level in a sinking ship and declaring everything seaworthy, while ignoring the twenty pumps running flat out to keep it afloat.

This hidden state, normal sugar paired with dangerously high insulin, can persist for ten, fifteen, even twenty years before the system finally begins to collapse and you get a diabetes diagnosis. But during those silent decades, the excess insulin is already driving disease. Already feeding cancer cells. Already damaging your brain. Already hardening your arteries. Already making you fatter and more resistant, year after year, in a vicious cycle that no amount of calorie counting can break.

What You're About to Learn

This book picks up where *The Fibre First Diet* left off.

In the chapters ahead, you will learn exactly how excess insulin drives cancer, through growth factor pathways that pharmaceutical drugs have been trying and failing to block for decades. You will understand why Alzheimer's is increasingly called type 3 diabetes, and what that means for your brain. You will see how heart disease is not primarily a cholesterol problem but an insulin problem, and why the medical establishment has been looking at the wrong blood marker for half a century.

You will also discover something that may surprise you: that the immune system most people never think about, the one powered by your gut, your bile, and a substance called taurine, is being systematically stripped by the very dietary advice we're told to follow.

And you will learn about GLP-1: what the weight loss injections actually do, what they miss, and how your body can produce this remarkable hormone naturally. Without a needle, without the side effects, and without the devastating muscle loss that these drugs are now known to cause.

I have written this book in plain English. Where Isabella explains a complex biological pathway, I will translate it into language anyone can understand. Where Ben presents research data, I will tell you what it means for your breakfast tomorrow morning. The science is real and rigorous. The language is human.

Because this information is too important to be locked behind medical terminology. It belongs to everyone.

• • •

A Note Before We Begin

I am not a doctor. I am not a biochemist. I am a sixty-year-old entrepreneur who became obese, watched his parents develop type 2 diabetes and Alzheimer's, and decided to do something about it. I have spent the last decade reading, researching, interviewing the world's leading scientists, writing six books, and putting much of what I've learned into practice on my own body.

At sixty, I am healthier, stronger, and sharper than I was at forty. Not because I'm special. Because I now know the truth.

That same truth is now in your hands. Let's begin.

CHAPTER TWO

Meet the Scientists

• • •

Before we go any further, I want to tell you about the two people whose scientific expertise shaped this book more than anyone else. You have already seen their names on the cover. I have been fortunate to learn from many brilliant people over the years, and I am grateful to every one of them. But when it came to understanding the deep science behind insulin resistance, it was Dr Isabella Cooper and Professor Ben Bikman who filled the gaps that I, as a businessman, could never have filled alone.

• • •

Dr Isabella Cooper

Isabella holds a first-class honours degree in Biochemistry with Medical Physiology, with advanced studies in cancer biology, endocrinology, immunology, and neurology. She is a member of the Royal Society of Biology, the Endocrine Society, the Biochemical Society, and the Physiological Society. She is an Associate Fellow of the Higher Education Academy and sits on the Scientific Advisory Board of the European Keto Live Centre. She has won multiple awards for scientific and teaching excellence, including Faculty of Science and Technology Awards and a UK Biochemical Society Award.

That is the formal version. Here is the version that matters more.

I first met Isabella at a health conference. I was presenting my *Tree of Afflictions* showing how insulin resistance connects to virtually every chronic condition. After my talk, this quietly brilliant scientist approached me and said, in effect, that I was right about the connections but that the mechanisms underneath were far more complex and far more damning than I had realised.

She was not being critical. She was being generous. And over the past year, through countless conversations, she patiently walked me through the biochemistry.

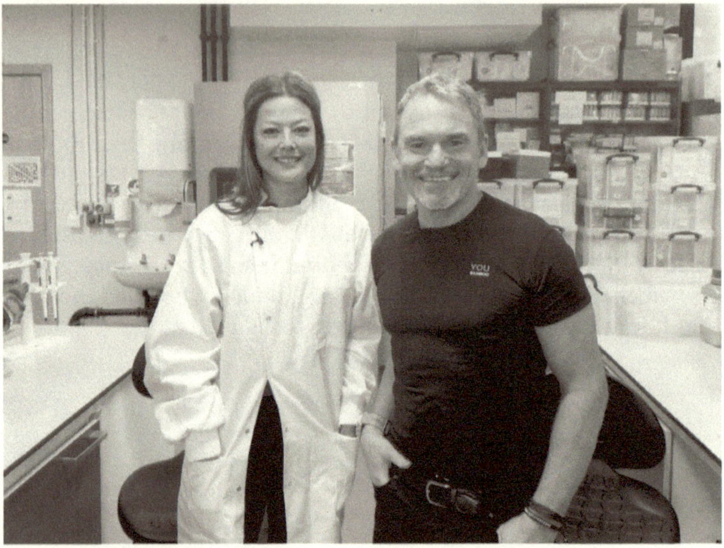

Visiting Isabella's laboratory at the University of Westminster

Isabella is half Chinese, and she brings a fascinating dual perspective to health science. On one side, there is her rigorous Western biochemistry training. On the other, there is a deep understanding of traditional Chinese dietary practices, things like fasting and bone broth as remedial foods, knowledge that has been passed down for thousands of years and is only now being validated by modern research.

She became deeply invested in health science through motherhood. The questions that pregnancy raised about nutrition, hormones, and the health of her children drove her deeper into the research than any academic career path alone would have done. That personal motivation, wanting to protect her own daughters, gives her work an urgency and honesty that you simply do not find in research funded by pharmaceutical companies.

Which brings me to the most important thing about Isabella: her research is entirely self-funded.

Her landmark study, the KetoSAge trial, was paid for out of her own pocket. No pharmaceutical company. No food industry sponsor. No government grant with strings attached. Just a scientist obsessed with finding the truth, in the old-fashioned sense of what a PhD is supposed to mean. And it didn't come cheap — this research cost around half a million pounds!

The KetoSAge study is one of the most remarkable pieces of research I have ever come across, and we will return to it several times in this book. In simple terms, Isabella took a group of healthy women who had been living in ketosis for an average of nearly four years. She measured everything: blood markers, hormones, growth factors, liver function, body composition, the lot. Then she asked them to follow the UK government's Eatwell Guide for just twenty-one days. Not junk food. Not fast food. Just the food our government tells us to eat.

The results were devastating. In three weeks, their insulin spiked. Their *IGF-1*, a growth factor strongly linked to cancer, tripled. Their natural *GLP-1* production, the very hormone that weight loss injections are trying to replace, dropped dramatically. Their liver markers worsened. When they went back to their normal ketogenic diet, everything reversed.

Twenty-one days on government guidelines. That is all it took to produce measurable damage in healthy people.

She is not just a collaborator. She is a friend. And the science she has shared with me, which I will do my best to translate for you in this book, is some of the most important work being done in metabolic health anywhere in the world.

• • •

Professor Ben Bikman

Ben Bikman is a professor of cell biology and physiology at Brigham Young University in the United States, and one of the world's leading experts on the role of insulin and fat cells in human health. His research laboratory focuses specifically on the metabolic origins of chronic disease, with particular emphasis on insulin resistance, obesity, and diabetes.

I first came across Ben through his books, which cut through the noise around insulin and metabolism in a way that very few scientists manage. His ability to explain complex biology in plain language reminded me of why I started writing my own books. I was so impressed that we invited him as a keynote speaker at our Public Health Collaboration conferences, not once but two years running. Since then, Ben has kindly given a great deal of his time for interviews with me and, along with Isabella, has volunteered to sit on my advisory panel at Clubwell.

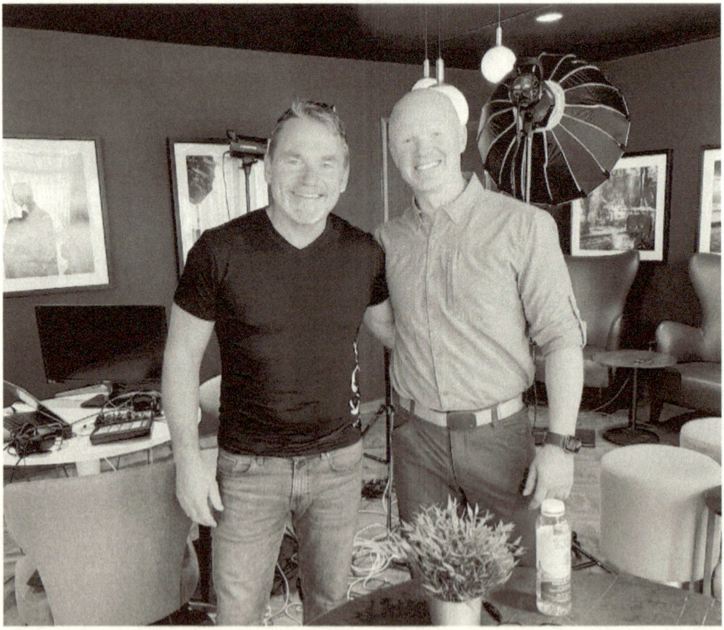

Ben and I backstage at the PHC Conference

In his laboratory at Brigham Young University, Ben and his students study fat cells. And one of my favourite things he ever told me was this. He can take fat cells in a petri dish and surround them with sugar, with energy, with calories, yet the fat cells will not grow at all. They simply cannot take up the energy. But add a tiny dash of insulin, and they soak it up like a sponge. That, in one simple experiment, tells you everything you need to know about what is really driving the obesity crisis. It is not the calories. It is the insulin.

Ben was also one of the earliest researchers to study the gut hormones that would later become the basis for weight loss injections like Ozempic and Wegovy. His PhD lab was at a medical school pioneering some of the first gastric bypass procedures, and his team was among the first funded in the United States to study incretin hormones, the family of gut hormones that includes GLP-1. He was there before GLP-1 even had a name.

As Ben explained to me:

"My dissertation lab was one of the first funded labs in the US to study the incretins, these gut hormones, because it was at a medical school where they were pioneering some of the earliest versions of the gastric bypass procedures. As the guts were being replumbed, that was leading to profound differences in GLP-1. It didn't even have a name yet."

That history gives Ben a unique perspective. He watched GLP-1 go from a research curiosity to a low-dose diabetes treatment to a high-dose weight loss phenomenon, and he has deep reservations about how it is being used today. We will explore those reservations in detail in Chapter 11.

Together, Isabella, Ben, and I co-authored a paper submitted to the House of Lords examining GLP-1 drugs and how to support people beyond them. The research behind that paper, combined with Isabella's groundbreaking KetoSAge study and Ben's decades of metabolic research, forms the scientific backbone of this book.

Why This Matters

I am not a scientist. I have said that already and I will say it again, because it matters. I am a businessman who built two companies to over a hundred million pounds and then walked away from it all to focus on health. A bit like the monk who sold his Ferrari, except I sold a gemstone empire and trained as a health coach. Not for money. Not for a second career. Just because I got fat, got furious about it, and decided that if I could figure this out for myself, I could help other people figure it out too. Along the way, I have been fortunate enough to meet and interview hundreds of doctors, researchers, authors, and health specialists. And among all of those brilliant people, two scientists in particular answered the questions I could not answer alone.

Isabella showed me the mechanisms. The pathways by which excess insulin drives cancer, destroys the brain, corrupts the immune system, and silently damages every organ in the body. She showed me the science behind the tree.

Ben showed me the metabolic trap. How calorie-restricted diets destroy your metabolism. How the very guidelines we are told to follow suppress the hormones that keep us healthy. And how the pharmaceutical industry is now selling us back, at enormous cost, something our bodies are perfectly capable of producing for free.

In the chapters that follow, I will bring their research to life in plain English. Where Isabella uses technical language, I will translate it. Where Ben presents data, I will tell you what it means for your next meal.

You deserve to know who is behind the science in this book. Now you do. Let's get into it.

CHAPTER THREE

The Insulin You Don't Know

• • •

In the last chapter, I introduced you to Isabella. Now I want to share one of the first things she said to me that reshaped how I think about health.

She told me that almost everything the public believes about insulin is wrong. Not slightly wrong. Fundamentally wrong.

Most people, if they think about insulin at all, think of it as the blood sugar hormone. The thing that diabetics inject. The thing your pancreas makes after you eat a biscuit. And yes, it does regulate blood sugar. We covered that in Chapter 1. But that is only a tiny fraction of what insulin actually does.

As Isabella explained it to me: insulin is not just a glucose-disposal molecule. It is a signalling hormone. Its job is to tell your cells what to do with the energy that is available. Depending on the mix of fuel in your bloodstream, whether that is glucose, protein, fatty acids, or ketones, insulin sends different instructions to your cells. It is like a conductor standing in front of an orchestra, deciding which instruments play and which ones stay silent.

When insulin is low and stable, the orchestra plays a calm, restorative piece. Your cells go into repair mode. They clean up damaged parts, recycle old proteins, and remove broken mitochondria. This process has a name: *autophagy*. Think of it as your body's internal housekeeping service. It sweeps the floors, takes out the rubbish, and patches up anything that needs fixing.

When insulin spikes, the music changes completely. Now the orchestra is playing something loud and fast. Your cells switch into growth mode. They stop cleaning up and start building. They divide, proliferate, and make more of themselves. That is fine in short bursts. After a meal, after exercise, your body needs to build and repair muscle. Insulin goes up, does its job, comes back down, and the housekeeping crew gets back to work. The problem, and this is the critical insight, is what happens when insulin stays high too often.

• • •

The Goldilocks Hormone

Isabella describes insulin as a Goldilocks hormone. At normal levels, it is essential for life. You cannot survive without it. Type 1 diabetics, whose pancreas produces no insulin at all, will die without injections. Insulin is not the enemy. Let me be absolutely clear about that.

But there is a threshold. And once you cross it, insulin stops being helpful and starts being destructive. This is not a simple case of more being better or less being better. It is a completely different effect. Low insulin tells your cells to clean and repair. Chronically high insulin tells your cells to grow and divide, while simultaneously shutting down every safety system that is supposed to keep that growth in check.

Imagine a factory with a production line and a quality control department. When things are running normally, the production line makes products and the quality control team checks them, catches defects, and pulls faulty items off the line. Now imagine the factory owner comes in and says: double production, triple production, run the machines twenty-four hours a day. And by the way, send the quality control team home. We do not have time for inspections.

That is what chronically elevated insulin does to your cells. It ramps up production and fires the quality control department. And the quality control department, in biological terms, is the system that catches and destroys damaged cells before they become dangerous. Before they become cancerous.

• • •

The Fat Trap

There is a piece of this story that we need to understand before we go any further, because it explains why so many people struggle to lose weight no matter how hard they try.

We know that insulin pushes glucose into muscle cells and liver cells, where it is either burned for energy or stored as glycogen. But insulin does not stop there. It also signals your fat cells to take it in. The difference is that fat cells do not use glucose for fuel. They use it to build something called *glycerol-3-phosphate*, which is essentially the scaffolding that holds fat molecules together. Think of it as the frame of a parcel. Without it, fat cannot be packaged and stored.

Now here is the second pathway, and this is the bigger one. When the liver gets more glucose than it can handle, it starts converting that excess into fatty acids through a process called *de novo lipogenesis*, which literally means "new fat creation." The liver then wraps those fatty acids into bundles called *triglycerides* and ships them out into your bloodstream. These bundles need somewhere to go. And insulin makes sure they get there. It activates an *enzyme* called *lipoprotein lipase* sitting on the surface of your fat cells, which cracks open those triglyceride bundles, pulls the fatty acids out, and feeds them straight into the cell for storage.

So, insulin is filling your fat cells from two directions at once. Glucose goes in to build the frame. Triglycerides go in to fill it up.

But here is the part that really matters. Insulin also does a third thing. It blocks the exit.

There is another enzyme called *hormone-sensitive lipase* whose entire job is to break down stored fat and release it back into the bloodstream so your body can burn it for energy. When insulin levels are high, this enzyme is suppressed. Switched off. Which means that while insulin is actively stuffing your fat cells from both sides, it is simultaneously locking the door so that none of that stored fat can ever get out. Isabella explains it simply:

"When insulin is elevated, your body is in storage mode. It is taking energy in, packing it away, and refusing to let any of it back out. That is why calorie restriction alone so often fails. You can eat less and less, but if insulin remains high, your body simply cannot access its own fat stores. You are starving in the middle of plenty."

Another colleague of mine, Professor Robert Lustig, is a paediatric endocrinologist (a doctor who specialises in diagnosing and treating hormone imbalances in children). For years he has helped obese children lose weight, not by counting calories, but by managing their hormones.

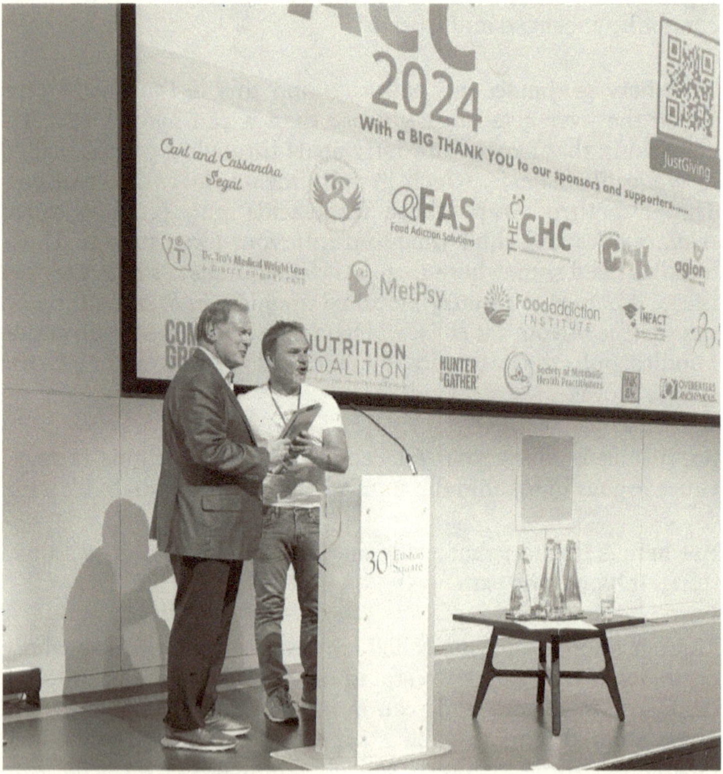

Presenting Robert with the Lifetime Achievement Award at the International Food Addiction Consensus Conference

Robert told me, "I realized that insulin was the bad guy and so we started changing what we did in clinic. Instead of worrying about weight, we worried about insulin. We said, get the insulin down any way you can, and that's what my clinic became. It became an insulin reduction clinic. It wasn't a weight loss clinic. It was an insulin reduction clinic, and when we got the insulin down, then they lost weight."

This is why people with chronically high insulin can diet for months, exercise every day, and barely lose a pound. It is not a lack of willpower. It is not laziness. It is biochemistry. The entrance to every fat cell is wide open and the exit is bolted shut.

The good news is that this works in reverse. When you bring insulin down, by eating fibre first, or by reducing processed carbohydrates (especially if you can get into ketosis), or by fasting, the exit unlocks. And your body finally gets permission to use the energy it has been hoarding for years.

This is exactly why ketosis matters, and why Isabella, Ben, and I talk about it so often. In ketosis, insulin is low. When insulin is low, all three of those mechanisms reverse.

1. ***Lipoprotein lipase*** on the outside of your fat cells quiets down, so triglycerides passing through the bloodstream are no longer being dragged into storage.

2. ***Hormone-sensitive lipase*** switches back on, so stored fat inside cells is finally being broken down and released as free fatty acids.

3. Your liver picks up these newly released fatty acids and converts them into ***ketones***, which your brain, heart, and muscles can burn for fuel.

Your fat cells go from being a one-way dumping ground to being your primary energy source. The door that insulin had bolted shut is wide open, and energy is flowing out instead of in. That is why measuring ketones in your blood, breath, or urine is so powerful. It is not just a number on a monitor. It is proof that the fat trap has been sprung.

No Insulin, Nobody Gets Fat

If everything I have just described sounds theoretical, let me give you the most powerful proof I know. Ben Bikman once told me that you could take a person, give them every other hormone in the human body, feed them tens of thousands of calories a day, and if you simply removed one single hormone, it would be completely impossible for that person to get fat. Not difficult. Not unlikely. Impossible.

That hormone is insulin.

He was not exaggerating. He was describing what happens every single day to people with type 1 diabetes.

In type 1 diabetes, the immune system destroys the beta cells in the pancreas that produce insulin. Without insulin injections, these people cannot store fat. It does not matter how much they eat. Their fat cells have no instruction to grow, so they do not grow. In fact, before insulin was discovered as a treatment, one of the telltale signs of type 1 diabetes was dramatic, unstoppable weight loss. The ancient physicians thought the body's flesh was turning to liquid and leaving through the urine. That is how powerful the absence of insulin is.

When a person with type 1 diabetes begins insulin therapy, they start gaining fat. Some patients gain so much weight in the first few days of treatment that they cannot leave the hospital in the clothes they arrived in. Nothing else changed. Same person, same diet, same body. The only difference was insulin.

This phenomenon is so well understood that it has created a formal eating disorder called diabulimia. Ben explains: Imagine a young woman, say thirteen years old, who is diagnosed with type 1 diabetes. Before her diagnosis, she could eat whatever she wanted and stay extremely thin. She liked that. Then she starts insulin injections and the weight begins to pile on. She learns that if she deliberately underdoses her insulin, she can eat anything she wants and stay as slim as she pleases. It works. It is devastatingly effective. And it is devastatingly dangerous, because without proper insulin, her body is slowly destroying itself. But the fact that diabulimia exists at all is absolute proof that fat storage is not simply a matter of calories in and calories out. It is a matter of insulin.

As I have already mentioned, in his laboratory, Ben and his students grow fat cells in petri dishes. These cells are sitting in a little sea of calories, surrounded by glucose and fats, everything a fat cell could possibly need to grow. And yet they stay small. They just sit there, doing nothing. The moment his team adds insulin to that petri dish, within four hours the cells are visibly fatter. Four hours later, fatter still. The calories were always there. The fat cells were always there. But without insulin, nothing happened. The cells did not know what to do with the energy around them until insulin arrived and gave the order.

This is not a theory. This is not a hypothesis waiting to be tested. This is observable, repeatable science happening in laboratories right now. And it tells us something that the calorie-counting industry does not want you to hear: you cannot get fat without insulin telling your fat cells to grow. Control your insulin, and you control the fate of your fat.

• • •

Not All Insulin Resistance Is Bad

Everything in this book so far has been about pathological insulin resistance, the kind that makes you sick. But there is another kind, and it is worth understanding the difference.

Your body deliberately creates insulin resistance twice during a normal human life. Ben Bikman calls them the two Ps: puberty and pregnancy.

During puberty, a child needs explosive growth. Bones, muscles, organs, everything expanding at once. Insulin is the body's growth signal, its fertiliser, and so the body temporarily raises insulin resistance to keep insulin levels high and fuel that growth.

It is physiological insulin resistance, meaning it is supposed to happen.

During pregnancy, the same thing occurs. A woman's body becomes insulin resistant on purpose, to grow the placenta, the uterus, the breast tissue, and to ensure extra glucose reaches the baby. Her body is also storing more fat as a safety net, an energy reserve in case food becomes scarce during the nine months. This is why pregnant women naturally gain weight. It is insulin doing exactly what evolution designed it to do.

The problem comes when physiological tips into pathological. If a pregnant woman already has a family history of type 2 diabetes, or if she is eating large amounts of sugar and refined carbohydrates throughout her pregnancy, her insulin resistance can go too far. At that point, her body can no longer keep glucose in check, and she is diagnosed with gestational diabetes, which is essentially type 2 diabetes of pregnancy.

And the consequences do not stop with her. Her baby develops in a high-sugar, high-insulin environment and gets hardwired to expect it. Research shows that children born to mothers with gestational diabetes have a 40% higher chance of becoming obese and developing metabolic complications in their teenage years and beyond.

• • •

Where Insulin Resistance Begins (And a Little About Fructose)

Professor Robert Lustig has spent over twenty-five years researching insulin and obesity. He has published hundreds of papers. He turned his obesity clinic into what he calls an "insulin reduction clinic." And his message is unambiguous: the roots of insulin resistance are in your liver.

Here is how. Your liver is a remarkable organ. It weighs about one and a half kilograms and it performs over 500 functions. But one of its most important jobs is acting as your body's metabolic gatekeeper. The liver gets first pass at most things you consume. It decides what to store, what to process, what to send on, and what to break down.

In this book we are focusing on how insulin resistance is driven in the main by too much glucose. But there is another sugar that has an equally devastating effect, just through a slightly different pathway. Fructose is the sweet molecule you find in a lot of fruit. It is also half of table sugar, which is 50% glucose and 50% fructose, and according to research by Robert fructose is added to roughly 73% of all products in the grocery store.

Unlike glucose, which can be used by every cell in your body, fructose can only be processed by the liver. It never gets into the bloodstream. Think about it: we have blood glucose monitors but not fructose monitors, because fructose never travels in the blood. It arrives at the liver in a flood, bypassing the normal feedback mechanisms that regulate glucose metabolism, and the liver has no choice but to deal with it.

When there is more fructose than the liver can handle, and in the modern diet there almost always is, the liver converts the excess directly into fat through *de novo lipogenesis*. Those fat molecules, triglycerides, begin to accumulate inside the liver cells. Some are exported into the bloodstream as *VLDL* particles, but much of the fat stays put, lodged inside the liver itself.

This is the beginning of fatty liver disease. And it does not take much. Robert points out that while you need to gain roughly ten kilograms of subcutaneous fat (the kind under your skin) before it causes metabolic problems, and about two kilograms of visceral belly fat, you need only a quarter of a kilogram of liver fat. Half a pound. That is all it takes to start breaking the system.

Once that fat accumulates, the liver cells become insulin resistant. They stop responding properly to insulin's signal to stop producing glucose. So, your liver keeps pumping glucose into your bloodstream even when it should not be, and your fasting blood sugar starts to creep up. Your pancreas detects this and does what it is designed to do: it produces more insulin. Louder knocking on a door that has stopped opening.

But there is a second problem happening at the same time that most people never hear about. A healthy liver clears about half the insulin that passes through it on that first pass from the pancreas. A fatty liver loses this ability. Its clearance drops. So now you have a pancreas that is producing more insulin than it should, and a liver that is failing to remove as much of it as it should. The result is a double hit. Systemic insulin levels rise far higher than they would in a healthy body.

And this is the point where the cascade becomes unstoppable. That chronically elevated insulin does not just affect the liver. It drives fat storage across the entire body. It amplifies every growth signal we discussed in the cancer chapter. It damages the blood-brain barrier. It triggers inflammation. It suppresses *SHBG*. It feeds every branch on the tree.

All of it traceable back to a fatty liver. All of it starting with too much sugar arriving too fast at an organ that was never designed to handle it in these quantities.

Robert puts it bluntly: "Fix the liver and you fix the problem." Because if the liver is where insulin resistance begins, then the liver is where the reversal must begin too. Stop flooding it with fructose and glucose. Give it a chance to clear the accumulated fat. Let it start doing its job again. And the entire cascade, from the pancreas to the fat cells to the brain to the immune system, begins to unwind.

• • •

Insulin's Second Message

To understand what happens next, you need to know about two pathways inside your cells. They both are master regulators that signal the cell to metabolise, grow, proliferate, to regulate homeostasis. I am going to give you their names, because you will see them again in this book, but do not worry about memorising them. Just understand what they do.

The first is called *m*TOR. It stands for mechanistic target of rapamycin (although for many years the "*m*" stood for mammalian), which is a mouthful, so let's just call it *m*TOR. Think of it as a volume switch inside every cell in your body. Think of it as a type of enzyme that controls how active the cell is. When *m*TOR is turned up, the cell grows and divides. When *m*TOR is turned down, the cell stops growing and switches to repair mode.

In a healthy body, *m*TOR pulses. It goes up when you eat, when you exercise, when your body needs to build muscle or heal a wound. Then it comes back down, and during that quiet period, the cell does its housekeeping. When turned down, it runs autophagy (the word literally translates to "self-eating," which is your body's way of digesting and recycling its own damaged parts), clears out cellular debris, repairs DNA, and checks itself for errors. This pulsing, up and down, growth and repair, is how a healthy cell is supposed to work.

Now here is the problem. When insulin is chronically elevated, *m*TOR gets stuck in the on position. It never comes down. The cell never gets a chance to do its housekeeping. It is building, building, building, all the time, with no quality checks, no repairs, and no error correction. That is a very dangerous state for a cell to be in. And it is the state that millions of people are living in every single day without knowing it.

The second is called the *PI3K/Akt* Pathway *(phosphoinositide 3-kinase / protein kinase B (Akt)*. Again, do not worry about the name. What matters is what it does. This pathway is triggered directly by insulin's growth signal. When insulin arrives at a cell and binds to its receptor (called RTKs – receptor tyrosine kinase), PI3K/Akt switches on and sends a clear instruction: proliferate. Make more of yourself.

Here is the twist that Isabella explained to me, and it took a while for it to sink in. When we talk about insulin resistance, we tend to think that the cells have stopped responding properly to insulin. That is true for glucose uptake. The cells are resisting to take a full load of sugar. But they have not stopped responding to insulin's growth signal. In fact, the opposite is true. Insulin-resistant cells become hypersensitive to the growth signal. They are ignoring the instruction to take up glucose, but they are amplifying the instruction to grow and divide. In Isabella's words:

"The cells have insulin receptors for glucose and also insulin receptors for growth, division, which lead to apoptosis inhibition."

We will mention it later but let me just quickly state that *apoptosis* is natural cell death, which is normally a good thing.

So, insulin is sending multiple messages to the cell at the same time: take in glucose and grow and divide. In a healthy person, both messages are received in proportion and everything runs smoothly. But to understand what goes wrong in insulin resistance, we need to look more closely at how glucose actually gets into the cell.

Both your muscle and fat cells have two types of glucose transporter on their surface. GLUT1 receptors are always present and always open. They provide a constant trickle of glucose for the cell's basic needs, no insulin required. GLUT4 receptors are different. They only move to the cell surface when insulin tells them to. *GLUT4* is activated after eating (postprandial), allowing a much larger surge of glucose in. It is the *GLUT4* receptors that stop responding in insulin resistance.

When a cell becomes insulin resistant, it stops translocating *GLUT4* receptors to its surface, which means it is no longer responding to insulin's instruction to take in extra glucose. But the cell is not starved of glucose entirely. It is still taking in its normal background supply through *GLUT1* receptors, which sit permanently on the cell surface and do not need insulin at all. The cell is getting enough glucose to function. What it has done is stopped listening to one specific part of insulin's message.

And here is what makes this so dangerous. At the very same time that the cell is refusing to open the *GLUT4* doors for glucose, it is responding even more aggressively to insulin's command to grow and divide. It is resistant to the useful part of insulin's message, and hypersensitive to the dangerous part. That is not a small detail. That is the mechanism by which insulin resistance drives cancer, and we will return to it in Chapter 4.

• • •

The Growth Factor Cascade

Insulin does not act alone. It is the first domino in a cascade of growth factors that, when chronically elevated, create the perfect conditions for disease.

The most important of these is called *IGF-1*, which stands for insulin-like growth factor 1. The name tells you a lot. It is a growth factor that looks and behaves like insulin, and insulin directly controls how much of it your body produces. More insulin means more IGF-1. In the KetoSAge study, when Isabella's participants switched from a ketogenic diet to the UK government's Eatwell Guide, their IGF-1 levels roughly tripled in just twenty-one days.

IGF-1 is a powerful promoter of cell growth. In the right context, at the right levels, it is perfectly healthy. Children need it to grow. When you hit the gym, you need it to build muscle. But when it is chronically elevated by persistently high insulin, it becomes a relentless growth signal that never switches off. And it does not just promote normal growth. It promotes the growth of any cell that has receptors for it, including damaged cells, precancerous cells, and cancer cells themselves.

But it gets worse. Insulin also controls how many IGF-1 receptors your cells produce. So not only does high insulin increase the amount of IGF-1 floating around in your blood, but it also increases the number of docking stations on your cells where IGF-1 can land and deliver its growth signal. And on top of that, insulin reduces the binding proteins that are supposed to regulate IGF-1 and keep it in check.

And here is a detail that really unsettled me when Isabella first explained it. IGF-1 and insulin can activate *each other's* receptors. They cross-activate. So even if you could somehow block one of them, the other would pick up the slack. This is why pharmaceutical drugs designed to target a single growth factor in cancer treatment have been so disappointing. As Isabella put it: they work beautifully in isolation, in a test tube, but in the real body, the other growth factors simply compensate.

• • •

The Hidden Damage

Now let me tell you why all of this is so dangerous, and why most people have absolutely no idea it is happening to them.

Your doctor, if they are checking your metabolic health at all, is almost certainly measuring your blood sugar. Perhaps your *HbA1c*, which gives an average of your blood sugar over the past three months. If those numbers come back normal, you are sent home with a clean bill of health.

But as we discussed in Chapter 1, you can have perfectly normal blood sugar while your insulin is through the roof. The sugar looks fine because the insulin is working overtime to keep it down. Your doctor is checking the water level in the ship and declaring it seaworthy, while twenty pumps are running flat out below deck.

Isabella calls this state "insulin-compensated euglycemia". In plain English, it means your blood sugar is normal, but only because your insulin is doing all the heavy lifting. And during those years, sometimes decades, of hidden high insulin, the damage is already happening. *m*TOR is stuck on. Autophagy is shut down. IGF-1 is elevated. Growth signals are flooding your cells. The quality control department has been sent home.

This is what Isabella calls the "little fires" mechanism. Excess insulin triggers constant, low-level damage throughout the body.

Inflammation. Oxidative stress. Mitochondrial dysfunction. Your body is continuously putting out these small fires with its repair systems, but when the fires never stop, the repair systems eventually get overwhelmed. And that is when disease takes hold.

This is why these diseases can also appear in people who are not overweight. We have been conditioned to think that cancer, heart disease, and Alzheimer's are diseases of obesity. They are not. They are diseases of elevated insulin. You can be slim and have dangerously high insulin. You can have normal blood sugar and still be on the path to cancer, because nobody has ever measured the thing that actually matters most. Insulin.

• • •

The Conductor in Your Cells

There is one more piece of this puzzle that I want to share with you before we move on to the specific diseases, and it is perhaps the most important of all.

Inside every cell in your body are tiny structures called *mitochondria*. You may remember them from school biology as the "powerhouses of the cell." They produce energy. That is true, but it is a bit like saying the conductor of the London Symphony Orchestra holds a stick. Technically correct, but it misses the point entirely.

Mitochondria are not just energy producers. They are the conductors of cellular behaviour. They decide what fuel the cell burns. They determine whether the cell grows or repairs. They control whether a damaged cell lives or dies. They are, in many ways, the decision-makers inside most of your thirty-seven trillion cells. And insulin controls them.

When insulin is low and you are burning fat or ketones for fuel, your mitochondria function beautifully. They produce energy cleanly, they manage their waste products properly, and they keep the cell in good working order. When insulin is chronically high and you are constantly burning glucose, the mitochondria come under stress. They produce too many waste products called *reactive oxygen species* (ROS). They start to malfunction. And when mitochondria malfunction, everything downstream goes wrong.

Isabella describes mitochondrial disruption as a common thread linking many chronic diseases. Cancer, Alzheimer's, heart disease, diabetes, autoimmune conditions. All of them, at their root, involve mitochondria that have stopped working properly. And the thing that is damaging those mitochondria, upstream of everything else, is chronically elevated insulin. As she put it to me:

"Insulin is the upstream mover and everything else is flowing downwards from it."

The interesting thing here is that if you listen to Professor Robert Lustig, you will often hear him say that ROS is the link to virtually all chronic disease. And if you listen to Isabella, she will tell you it is dysfunctional mitochondria. You could argue they are both right. But what comes first? What causes the ROS? What damages the mitochondria? Elevated insulin. It is always the insulin.

• • •

Why This Changes Everything

If you take one thing from this chapter, let it be this. Insulin is not just the blood sugar hormone. It is the master controller of growth, repair, and cellular behaviour. When it is working properly, pulsing up and down in response to meals and activity, it keeps your body in balance. Growth when you need it. Repair when you need it. A well-run factory with a production line and a quality control department working in harmony.

But when insulin stays elevated, day after day, year after year, it flips a switch. Growth without repair. Production without quality control. A cascade of growth factors with nothing to keep them in check. And the damage builds silently, invisibly, for years or even decades before it shows up as a diagnosis.

In the chapters that follow, we are going to look at exactly how this plays out in the diseases that are destroying millions of lives. We will start with the one that frightens people most, and the one where Isabella's research is most groundbreaking: cancer.

But before we go there, I want you to remember something. This is not a book about fear. It is a book about understanding. Because once you understand the mechanism, you also understand how to stop it. And stopping it is far simpler than the pharmaceutical industry would have you believe.

I find that comforting, and I hope you will too. It would be easy to read a book like this and feel overwhelmed. Cancer. Alzheimer's. Heart disease. Diabetes. A list like that can make you feel like you are walking through a minefield, waiting for the next one to get you. Especially if you are the sort of person who lies awake at night worrying about your health.

But here is what I want you to take from these pages. These diseases are not random. They are not bad luck. They are not inevitable. Remember, virtually all of them were unheard of 150 years ago. They have a cause, and that cause is something you can measure, understand, and change. That is not frightening. That is empowering.

CHAPTER FOUR

How Insulin Causes Cancer

• • •

This is the chapter I have been building towards. Through my conversations with Ben Bikman, and a great deal of research for *The Fibre First Diet*, I had come to understand the link between insulin and certain cancers. Breast cancer and colon cancer, in particular, made sense to me. The mechanisms were relatively straightforward, and the research was compelling. But I struggled to comprehend how insulin could be driving so many other types of cancer. The connections felt real, but I could not see the pathways clearly enough to explain them. That is where Isabella truly enlightened me. She showed me that the link between insulin and cancer is not a vague association or a statistical correlation. It is a set of specific, biological pathways that, once you understand them, change the way you think about this disease forever.

I want to be upfront about something. This chapter contains more science than any other in this book. I have done my best to keep it in plain English, and I will translate every technical term as we go; the glossary will probably prove to be invaluable too. But the science matters here, because for too long people have been told that cancer is just bad luck, or bad genes, or something that randomly happens to unlucky people. It is not. In a great many cases, cancer is the predictable result of a metabolic environment that allows it to grow. And the single biggest driver of that environment is chronically elevated insulin.

• • •

Cancer Cells Are Not What You Think

Let me start by clearing up a common misunderstanding. Most people think of cancer as a genetic disease. A mutation happens in your DNA, a cell goes rogue, and it starts dividing out of control. That is partly true. Mutations do play a role. But the question nobody seems to ask is: why do some mutated cells become cancer, while others are caught and destroyed by the body before they ever cause a problem?

The answer is that your body has a surveillance system. Every single day, your immune system identifies and destroys damaged cells, precancerous cells, and cells with DNA errors. It does this through a process called *apoptosis*, which is programmed cell death. Think of it as your body's quality control system. When a cell is damaged beyond repair, it receives a signal to self-destruct. It quietly takes itself apart, gets recycled, and is replaced by a healthy cell. This happens millions of times a day without you ever knowing about it.

Cancer does not happen because a cell mutates. Cancer happens when that quality control system fails. When damaged cells are allowed to survive, divide, and grow, because the signals that should have told them to self-destruct have been switched off.

And what switches those signals off? Chronically elevated insulin.

There is a remarkable experiment that proves this is a metabolic problem, not a genetic one, and I want to share it with you because it changes the way you think about cancer entirely.

A scientist called Dr Thomas Seyfried did something beautifully simple. He took the nucleus from a cancer cell, the part that contains all the DNA, all the genes, all the mutations that we have been told cause cancer, and he placed it inside a healthy cell. If cancer were truly a genetic disease, that cell should have become cancerous. It had the cancer's DNA. It had every mutation. And yet the cell remained completely normal. It did not become cancerous at all.

Then he did the opposite. He took the mitochondria from the cancer cell, the tiny energy factories, and placed them into a healthy cell. It became cancerous.

Think about what that means. The DNA did not matter. The mutations did not matter. What mattered was the mitochondria, the part of the cell that controls how energy is processed. When the energy system was broken, the cell became cancerous. When the energy system was healthy, even cancer DNA could not make it cancerous.

This is why Ben Bikman, Isabella Cooper, Thomas Seyfried, and a growing number of researchers now see cancer not as a disease of bad genes, but as a disease of broken metabolism. And what breaks your cellular metabolism more than anything else? Insulin.

• • •

The Receptors on the Door

In the last chapter, I explained how insulin, beyond managing blood sugar levels, is a signalling hormone that tells cells to grow and divide. Now I want to show you exactly how that plays out in cancer, because the mechanisms are far more sophisticated and far more alarming than most people realise.

As we have already discussed, every cell in your body has receptors on its surface. Think of them as locks on a door. Different hormones and growth factors act as keys. When the right key fits the right lock, a signal is sent inside the cell telling it what to do.

Normal cells have insulin receptors. Cancer cells have many times more. They are covered in these receptors. That means cancer cells are vastly more sensitive to insulin's growth signal than the healthy cells around them. Every time insulin levels rise, cancer cells hear that signal louder and more clearly than any other cell in your body.

In 1989, a team led by Pezzino and Vigneri published a study that put hard numbers on this. They measured insulin receptors directly in 159 breast cancer specimens and compared them with normal breast tissue. The cancer cells had more than six times the number of insulin receptors. Not a small increase. Six times. And those receptors were fully functional, binding insulin and activating growth signals exactly like normal receptors, only six times louder.

What does that mean in practice? Every time insulin arrives at one of those cells, six times as many receptors are picking up the signal. That means a louder instruction to open the glucose doors and a louder instruction to grow and divide. The cell is pulling in more fuel and receiving a stronger growth command at the same time.

The researchers also found that the more insulin receptors the tumour had, the larger it was and the more aggressive its grading. More receptors meant more insulin getting through. More insulin meant more glucose flooding in and a louder growth signal. A louder growth signal meant faster, more dangerous growth. The study even found that the insulin receptor content in these breast cancers was higher than in any normal tissue in the body, including the liver.

Now pause and think about what that means for a woman with chronically elevated insulin. Every time her insulin spikes, those cancer cells, if they exist, are hearing that growth signal six times louder than the healthy tissue around them. They are not just growing. They are growing faster than everything else in her body.

But insulin is not the only key turning these locks. As Isabella explained to me, insulin controls a whole cascade of growth factors, and every single one of them is involved in cancer progression.

Let me walk you through the main ones, but before I do let me explain about hyper-proliferative cells.

• • •

Hyper-Proliferative Cells

Here is where it gets really unsettling. When you become insulin resistant, your cells stop responding properly to insulin's instruction to take in glucose. That much we know. But here is the crucial part that most people miss: just because those cells have stopped listening to the glucose message does not mean they have stopped listening to insulin altogether. They are still receiving the insulin signal. They are just responding to a different part of it.

Certain cells in your body are what we call "hyper-proliferative." These are cells that naturally need to divide on a regular basis to keep your organs functioning. Your lungs, breast tissue, prostate, intestines, brain, kidneys, and liver all contain these rapidly dividing cells. It is simply how those tissues maintain themselves. Old cells die; new ones replace them. It is one of the most elegant systems in the human body.

But when insulin levels are chronically elevated, something dangerous happens. And it is not what you might expect.

In a healthy body, insulin sends two messages to these cells at the same time: take in glucose through *GLUT4* receptors and grow and divide through separate growth *pathways*. Both messages are received in proportion and everything runs smoothly.

In an insulin resistant body, the *GLUT4* glucose transporters stop responding. They no longer move to the cell surface, so the insulin-dependent door for extra glucose shuts down. But fast-growing cells (hyper-proliferative), the kind that become tumours, do not and cannot go hungry. They find another way in.

Through a chain reaction that Isabella has mapped in detail, chronically high insulin suppresses a protein in the liver called SHBG (sex hormone-binding globulin). When SHBG drops, the growth signals reaching these cells change. Their DNA expression shifts. And the result is remarkable: the cells start producing more *GLUT1* receptors and embedding them permanently in their membranes. *GLUT1* does not need insulin. It is always on. These cells have effectively installed a constant glucose tap that runs day and night, completely bypassing the lock that insulin resistance put on the front door.

Think of insulin as a bunch of keys. In a healthy body, those keys open all the right doors in the right order. But in an insulin resistant body, the *GLUT4* door is jammed. The key does not fit any more. So, the cell builds itself a new entrance, a permanently open *GLUT1* window that does not need a key at all. Glucose flows in around the clock.

Meanwhile, the growth signal works differently. It is not a door at all. It is more like an intercom on the outside of the house. Insulin presses the buzzer, and the message travels inside the cell: grow and divide. As insulin resistance develops and the *GLUT4* door jams shut, something dangerous happens. The growth intercom does not get quieter. It amplifies. The receiver inside the cell turns up the volume. So now you have a cell that is struggling to take in glucose through the normal front door but is receiving an ever-louder instruction to grow, divide, and ignore the off switch. The cell has unlimited fuel from *GLUT1* and an amplified growth signal from insulin. That is the perfect storm.

Now here is the really frightening part. Our bodies have never evolved a system that would tell a cell to grow and divide whilst simultaneously telling it to self-destruct. That would be biologically absurd. You would not build a house and demolish it at the same time. So, when insulin switches on the "grow" signal, it automatically switches off apoptosis, the mechanism by which damaged or worn-out cells are programmed to die in a controlled, orderly way.

And that, in simple terms, is how we define cancer. Cells that grow and divide too much and cannot die when they should.

So excess insulin (*hyperinsulinaemia*) is doing two things at once. It is forcing naturally proliferative cells to proliferate even faster. And it is preventing the very process that would normally keep them in check. The accelerator is jammed down and the brakes have been cut. Isabella explains how this situation progresses further:

"So, the more that apoptosis is switched off, the more damage and dysfunction inside of the cell happens, and that results not just in the potential for cancer, but in terms of the mitochondria becoming toxic, unhealthy, dysregulated, and doing a lot of other damage in the body that is not necessarily just cancer. Autoimmune conditions, dementia, and things like that."

• • •

IGF-1: The Growth Amplifier

We introduced *IGF-1*, insulin-like growth factor 1, in the last chapter. But its role in cancer deserves much deeper attention, because this is where things start to get truly alarming. Insulin directly controls how much *IGF-1* your body produces. More insulin means more *IGF-1*. In Isabella's KetoSAge study, when healthy women switched from a ketogenic diet to the UK government's Eatwell Guide, their IGF-1 levels tripled in just twenty-one days.

IGF-1 is one of the most potent growth promoters in the human body. It tells cells to grow, divide, and multiply. In the right context, that is perfectly healthy. But when it is chronically elevated, it sends that growth signal constantly, to every cell with a receptor for it. Including cancer cells.

And remember what I said about insulin receptors and *IGF-1* receptors being able to cross-activate each other? This means that even if you could somehow block the insulin receptor on a cancer cell, *IGF-1* would simply use its own receptor to deliver the same growth signal. And vice versa. The two systems are intertwined so deeply that blocking one without blocking the other is like plugging one hole in a sieve.

This is why pharmaceutical drugs designed to target *IGF-1* in cancer treatment have been so disappointing. They work well in a test tube, in isolation. But in the real human body, insulin compensates. The other growth factors compensate. The system finds a way around the blockade, because the underlying cause, the chronically elevated insulin, has not been addressed.

Isabella listed five of these growth factors by name, each one linked to cancer progression, and explained why blocking them individually has never worked:

"Every single one of them, VEGF, EGF, IGF-1, FGF, leptin, is involved in cancer progression. We have drug trials and drugs that are made to try and block one. But the problem is, with a drug to block for example VEGF, insulin can trigger VEGF's receptor. So, these drugs never seem to work really well, because in isolation, they're fantastic, but then in the wider picture in the real body, those other markers will cross-activate and trigger them."

Let me put that in plain English. The pharmaceutical industry has spent billions trying to block individual growth factors that drive cancer. But because insulin is upstream of all of them, and because they can all activate each other's receptors, blocking one is like cutting one head off a hydra. The others simply take over. The only way to turn them all down at once is to address the thing that is driving them all: the insulin.

• • •

The Kill Switch That Gets Turned Off

If the growth signal were the only problem, it would be bad enough. But insulin does something even more dangerous. It disables the system that is supposed to catch and destroy cancer cells before they can spread.

Inside every cell, there are two proteins of the same family locked in a constant tug of war. One is called *BCL-2*, which is a survival protein. Its job is to keep the cell alive. The other is called BAX, which is a death protein. Its job is to trigger apoptosis, the self-destruct sequence, when a cell is damaged.

In a healthy cell, these two are balanced. If the cell is healthy, *BCL-2* keeps it alive. If the cell is damaged, *BAX* tips the balance and the cell destroys itself. It is an elegant system that has been fine-tuned over millions of years of evolution.

But chronically elevated insulin tips this balance in favour of survival. It increases BCL-2 and suppresses *BAX*. The kill switch can get stuck in the off position. Damaged cells that should have been destroyed are instead allowed to survive. And those surviving damaged cells, amongst a few other causes, are the ones that go on to become tumours.

This happens through *SHBG*. As we saw a few pages ago, high insulin suppresses it. But *SHBG* does not just affect *GLUT1*. It also regulates *BCL-2*, the cell survival protein. When *SHBG* drops, *BCL-2* rises, and the cell's ability to self-destruct when damaged is compromised.

• • •

The Warburg Effect: How Cancer Cells Feed

In 1924, a Nobel Prize-winning scientist called Otto Warburg made a discovery. He found that cancer cells process glucose differently from normal cells. Instead of burning it cleanly in their mitochondria through a process called oxidative phosphorylation, cancer cells ferment glucose into lactate. They do this even when there is plenty of oxygen available. It is an incredibly wasteful way to produce energy, using far more glucose to generate far less fuel. But cancer cells do it anyway.

To understand why this matters, it helps to know what lactate is. In a healthy person, lactate is the waste product your muscles produce during intense exercise. It is the burn you feel when you sprint flat out or push through the last few repetitions of a heavy lift. Your muscles only resort to this when they are working so hard that oxygen delivery cannot keep up, so they switch to a faster, cruder way of producing energy called glycolysis. This process happens in the cytoplasm, outside the mitochondria, acting as an emergency backup, not the default setting. But cancer cells use this emergency backup all the time, even at rest, even when oxygen is plentiful. And because this process is so inefficient, they need to consume vastly more glucose than normal cells to keep going.

A normal cell can extract around 36 units of energy from a single glucose molecule. A cancer cell fermenting that same molecule into lactate gets just 2. That is why cancer cells are such ravenous consumers of sugar. They are running a factory on a system designed for emergencies.

For almost a century, scientists debated why cancer cells would choose something so wasteful. The answer, which Isabella walked me through in extraordinary detail, comes down to a switch inside the cell called HIF-1α. You do not need to remember the name. What matters is what it does. In a healthy cell, unless you're sprinting or lifting really heavy things, this switch stays off, and glucose is burned cleanly and efficiently in the mitochondria. Think of it as a clean furnace running smoothly.

But when HIF-1α gets turned on, often by low oxygen or abnormal signals from chronic insulin, it diverts glucose away from the mitochondria and into fermentation. The clean furnace gets shut down. The dirty, wasteful backup generator takes over. And the byproducts of that dirty process, including lactate and damaging molecules called *reactive oxygen species (ROS)*, cause even more harm to the cell, creating a vicious cycle. This is the Warburg effect: cancer cells stuck on the wrong fuel system, burning through enormous amounts of glucose and producing waste that makes everything worse.

Now here is where it comes full circle. Your body has a natural way to help keep the HIF-1α switch turned off: *melatonin*, the hormone your body produces when you sleep in the dark. But what undermines melatonin production? Disrupted sleep, light at night from screens and devices, and the metabolic chaos of chronically elevated insulin.

Let me repeat this again, as it is so important to grasp. In healthy cells under normal oxygen levels, HIF-1α stays off, allowing glucose to burn cleanly and efficiently through the Krebs cycle inside the mitochondria. It flips on only during stresses like hypoxia (where cells don't get enough oxygen to function properly) or intense sprinting (e.g., chasing a bus), transiently boosting glycolysis for rapid *ATP* production without fully shutting down mitochondria. This adaptive "flick" is temporary and beneficial.

In disease like cancer, however, chronic activation locks cells into wasteful fermentation (the Warburg effect), producing damaging lactate and reactive oxygen species in a vicious cycle. To help keep this switch off and favour healthy metabolism, prioritise good sleep for high melatonin production and work to reduce insulin resistance.

So, the same excess insulin that is sending growth signals, amplifying IGF-1, suppressing the kill switch through SHBG and BCL-2, and flooding cells with glucose through GLUT1, may also be disabling one of your body's natural brakes on the Warburg effect, all amplified by poor sleep. Every road leads back to insulin.

. . .

The PET Scan Proof

If you have ever known anyone who has had a PET scan for cancer, you may already know this next part. But it was Isabella who made me see its full significance. When you go for a PET scan, they inject you with something called FDG, which is a glucose analogue. Think of it as a fake glucose, a molecule that is so nearly identical to real glucose that your cells cannot tell the difference. It gets into cells through exactly the same doorways as real glucose. But here is the clever part: once inside, the cell cannot actually use it for fuel. It is a poser. It gets in but it goes nowhere. So, it just sits there, glowing on the scanner. And where does it accumulate most? In the cancer cells.

Because cancer cells are desperately hoarding glucose through all those extra GLUT1 receptors we just talked about, they drink up more FDG than any other tissue. The fake glucose lights them up like a Christmas tree on the scan. That is how your oncologist finds the tumour. Cancer's hunger for glucose is so intense that it betrays its own location.

Read that again. The very tool we use to detect cancer works by exploiting the fact that cancer cells are guzzling glucose faster than any other cell in the body.

And yet, despite using a glucose-based dye to detect cancer, mainstream medicine has been remarkably slow to ask the obvious question: what if we reduced the glucose supply to prevent and potentially stop cancer growth?

Here is another detail that shook me. Many people with early-stage cancer have perfectly normal HbA1c, the blood sugar marker your doctor checks. How is that possible if cancer cells are consuming so much glucose? Because the cancer is eating it, the tumour is acting like a glucose vacuum, sucking up so much sugar that your blood sugar levels look normal. Your doctor checks your HbA1c, sees a healthy number, and tells you everything is fine. Meanwhile, the reason it looks fine is that a tumour is consuming the evidence.

• • •

A Real-Life Story

One of the most powerful stories I have come across in all my research came from Dr Annette Bosworth, known as Dr Boz, an internal medicine physician from South Dakota. I was lucky enough to interview her on my podcast, and her story stopped me in my tracks.

Her mother, Grandma Rose, had been battling chronic lymphocytic leukaemia for years. She had been through two rounds of chemotherapy. The second round was so brutal it disconnected her brain from her body. This was a woman who had hand-sewn every piece of clothing her daughter wore until she was ten years old, and after chemo she could not tell you what a sewing machine did. It took six months to teach her brain to recover that single skill.

Then the numbers climbed again. The oncologist said she needed a third round. And Grandma Rose, grey-faced and exhausted, looked at her daughter and said, *"I am not doing that again. The clothes I want at my funeral are at the top of that closet in the basement."*

They walked out of the consulting room holding the referral slip. One corridor led to chemotherapy. The other led to the front door. And Grandma Rose asked the question that changed everything: *"If it was you, what would you do?"*

Dr Boz had recently stumbled across research on ketones and the brain, through a podcast between Dom D'Agostino and Tim Ferriss. She had been studying the ketogenic diet for neurological repair and had read just enough about the Warburg effect and cancer metabolism to know there might be something in it. She had no clinical evidence for this specific cancer. No protocol to follow. No published case study. But she looked at her mother and said, *"Mom, I would walk out that front door and do something called the ketogenic diet."*

They drove back to the farm together. Cleared every carbohydrate out of the house. Forty years of canned goods, gone. Dr Boz told her whole family, including her young children, that they were all going keto in the name of Grandma Rose. They sent each other photos of their ketone readings every morning. No half measures.

Six weeks later, Grandma Rose walked back into the oncologist's office. The staff drew her blood, then drew it again, convinced the samples had been mislabelled. The oncologist searched for chemotherapy records, certain she must have had treatment somewhere else. When he could not find them, he sat down and said, *"Well then, how did you lower your numbers by 70%?"*

No chemotherapy. No drugs. Just the removal of sugar and the production of ketones. Her colour had returned. Her energy was back. She had been on antibiotics for 50 out of the previous 52 weeks. She no longer needed them. And for the first time in years, Dr Boz could see a sparkle in her eyes.

When I asked Dr Boz what level of ketosis she aims for with her most serious patients, her answer was clear: get the blood ketone reading to roughly half of the blood glucose reading and hold it there. That is the therapeutic zone.

• • •

The Oestrogen Connection

We have already seen how insulin suppresses *SHBG* and the damage that causes. But in breast cancer, there is an additional pathway.

Isabella shared a fascinating observation with me. An eighteen-year-old girl has the highest oestrogen (if you're in America that's how we Europeans spell estrogen) levels she will ever have in her life. And yet eighteen-year-olds have among the lowest rates of breast cancer. A forty-five-year-old woman has lower oestrogen levels, but a significantly higher risk of breast cancer. If oestrogen itself were a primary driver of breast cancer, this would make no sense. The answer lies in *SHBG* (sex hormone-binding globulin).

At eighteen, SHBG levels are high. *SHBG* binds to oestrogen and changes the way it signals to cells. The *SHBG-oestrogen complex* produces a different, safer signalling cascade than free oestrogen alone. So even though the eighteen-year-old has more oestrogen, it is being properly regulated by *SHBG*.

By forty-five, after decades of elevated insulin from a modern diet, SHBG levels have dropped. Now the oestrogen, even though there is less of it, is signalling differently. Without SHBG to regulate it, the oestrogen signal becomes more potent and more dangerous. Combine that with elevated *IGF-1*, elevated *GLUT1*, suppressed apoptosis, and damaged mitochondria, and you have a perfect storm for cancer growth.

And the trigger for all of it? The same thing. Chronically elevated insulin.

• • •

*m*TOR: The Switch That Never Turns Off

We covered *m*TOR briefly in the last chapter, but in the context of cancer, it deserves more attention. In a healthy cell, *m*TOR pulses. It goes up during feeding and exercise, promoting growth and repair, then it comes back down, allowing the cell to run its housekeeping programmes: autophagy, DNA repair, error checking.

In a cancer cell, *m*TOR is permanently stuck in the on position. It never comes down. The cell is in permanent growth mode, permanently building, permanently dividing. And all of the housekeeping programmes that should be catching errors and clearing out damage? They have been shut down.

Think of it like a car factory that runs the production line twenty-four hours a day, seven days a week, while simultaneously firing every quality inspector, disconnecting every safety sensor, and ignoring every warning light on the dashboard. Cars are rolling off the line, but nobody is checking whether they work. Nobody is checking whether they are safe. And the ones that are defective are not being pulled from the line. They are being sent straight out into the world.

That is what *m*TOR does when it is stuck on. And what keeps *m*TOR stuck on? The PI3K/Akt pathway, which is triggered by insulin. Once again, the trail leads back to the same place.

• • •

Why the Drugs Keep Failing

I want to pause here and address something that may be forming in your mind. If all of these pathways are so well understood, why have we not cured cancer?

We have touched on this twice already in this chapter, first when we discussed how insulin cross-activates growth factor receptors, and again when we looked at how blocking one pathway simply pushes the signal through another. But it is important enough to pull together in one place, because it reveals something fundamental about the way we have been fighting this disease.

The pharmaceutical approach to cancer has been to target these pathways one at a time. There are drugs that block IGF-1. Drugs that inhibit *m*TOR. Drugs that target VEGF, the growth factor that builds blood vessels to feed tumours. In isolation, in a petri dish, many of these drugs work brilliantly.

But in the human body, they consistently underperform. And the reason is cross-activation. When you block VEGF, insulin can trigger VEGF's receptor through a different route. When you block IGF-1, insulin compensates through PI3K. When you block *m*TOR, the upstream signals simply find another way around. It is like trying to stop a river by blocking one tributary. The water just flows around the obstruction.

The pharmaceutical approach treats each growth factor as a separate target. But they are not separate. They are all downstream of the same thing. They are all amplified by the same hormone. And until you address that hormone, no single-target drug is going to completely solve the problem.

Isabella puts it plainly: excess insulin harms your mitochondria. And anything that chronically damages your mitochondria will increase uncontrolled cell proliferation and block apoptosis. That is the cancer phenotype.

It is especially dangerous in tissues that are naturally fast-dividing, what scientists call highly mitotic. These are cells that are already splitting into identical copies of themselves as part of their normal function: intestinal cells, prostate, breast, lung, liver, pancreas, and the glia cells in your brain. These tissues are already on the edge. Add damaged mitochondria to the mix, and the brakes come off entirely.

• • •

It Is Not Just Insulin

I want to be honest about something. Insulin resistance is, in my view, the single biggest driver of cancer that nobody talks about. It is the trunk of the tree. But it is not the only thing feeding the branches. There are other forces at work, and many of them are hiding in plain sight. What makes them doubly dangerous is that most of them also drive insulin resistance itself. They are not just separate risks. They feed the trunk.

Let's start with chronic stress. When you are stressed, your body pumps out cortisol. Cortisol raises blood sugar. Blood sugar triggers insulin. So chronic stress does not just make you feel awful, it keeps insulin elevated by the back door. But cortisol does more than that. It suppresses your immune system, the very system responsible for detecting and destroying rogue cells before they become tumours. If your body is in a permanent state of fight or flight, it is not doing its housekeeping. Cancer cells that would normally be caught and cleared get a free pass.

Then there are seed oils. Sunflower oil, rapeseed oil, soybean oil, safflower oil. They are found in virtually every processed food product on the supermarket shelf. These oils are loaded with omega-6 fatty acids, which in excess drive chronic inflammation. And as we have already discussed in this book, chronic inflammation is one of the key conditions that allows cancer to take hold and grow. In my previous books I have written in some detail about how the modern diet has pushed the omega-6 to omega-3 ratio from roughly 1:1, which is what our ancestors evolved on, to something closer to 20:1. That is not a minor imbalance. That is a metabolic environment primed for disease.

Lectins deserve a mention too. These are proteins found in certain plants, particularly grains, legumes, and nightshades, that can irritate the gut lining when consumed in large amounts. A damaged gut lining lets molecules through that should not get through, triggering immune responses and low-grade inflammation. Again, the same pattern: anything that drives chronic inflammation creates conditions that favour cancer growth.

Now consider the chemicals we are exposed to every day. BPA (bisphenol A) is found in plastic bottles, food packaging, and tin can linings. It is an endocrine disruptor, meaning it mimics oestrogen in your body. Research has shown that even low doses alter hormone-sensitive organs and are linked to a wide range of diseases. A recent study by the Center for Environmental Health found that sports bras and athletic shirts from major fast fashion brands contained BPA levels up to 40 times the safe limit. You are absorbing it through your skin, bypassing the liver entirely, straight into the bloodstream.

And it is not just BPA. Polyester and other synthetic fabrics contain PFAS, formaldehyde, and phthalates, all known endocrine disruptors. These chemicals interfere with your hormonal balance, and as we have seen throughout this book, hormonal disruption and insulin resistance feed each other. When oestrogen or testosterone is thrown out of balance by external chemicals, the knock-on effects reach every branch of the tree.

Even the air we breathe and the products we put on our skin contribute. As I wrote in *The Fibre First Diet*, what you apply to your skin bypasses your liver's gatekeeper function and goes directly into your bloodstream. If you would not eat it, think twice before rubbing it into your skin.

But here is the point I want to come back to, because it matters. Every single one of these factors, stress, seed oils, lectins, BPA, synthetic chemicals, does its worst damage in a body that is already metabolically compromised. They pour petrol on a fire that insulin resistance has already lit. In a metabolically healthy body with low insulin, functioning mitochondria, and a strong immune system, these insults can be better handled. Your body has the tools to neutralise them. But when insulin is chronically elevated, when your mitochondria are damaged, when your immune system is suppressed, these everyday exposures become genuinely dangerous. They do not cause cancer on their own. But in a body already primed by insulin resistance, they may accelerate it.

Fix the insulin first. Then you give your body the best possible chance of dealing with everything else.

• • •

What This Means for You

I know this chapter has been heavy. It is the hardest chapter in this book to comprehend, and I have deliberately not softened it, because I believe you deserve the truth. Cancer is not random. In a great many cases, it is the result of a metabolic environment that has been created by decades of chronically elevated insulin, driven by a diet that our own government recommends.

But here is the other side of this. If the environment drives the cancer, then changing the environment can help prevent it.

And the single most powerful thing you can do to change that environment is to manage your insulin.

Keep your insulin low, and you lower IGF-1. You allow SHBG to do its job. You restore the BCL-2/BAX balance so damaged cells can self-destruct as they should. You allow melatonin to suppress HIF-1α. You let *m*TOR pulse instead of staying permanently on. You turn down every growth factor in the cascade, not by blocking them one at a time with expensive drugs, but by removing the thing that is driving them all.

I want to be very clear here: none of this is medical advice. If you or a loved one is currently taking medication to manage cancer, please do not change anything based on what I have written. But perhaps use it to ask questions. What else could you be doing alongside your treatment? What conversations could you be having with your oncologist about diet, insulin, and metabolic health? Knowledge is not a replacement for medical care. It is a reason to demand the best medical care.

In the KetoSAge study, all of these markers improved when participants returned to a low-insulin lifestyle. In just twenty-one days. The same amount of time it took for the government guidelines to make them worse.

We will talk about exactly how to do this in the final chapters of this book. But first, we need to follow the trail of insulin's damage further, into the brain, the heart, and other parts of your body that you probably never connect to what you eat.

CHAPTER FIVE

How Insulin Causes Alzheimer's

• • •

This chapter is personal. More personal than any other in this book.

My parents met when they were fourteen years old. Teenagers who fell in love and stayed in love. They shared meals together for nearly seventy years, eating the same food, at the same table, day after day, decade after decade. A testament to their culinary compatibility, you might say. They both ate the same carbohydrate-heavy, traditional British diet that their generation was raised on.

My dad developed type 2 diabetes. My mum developed Alzheimer's.

Two different diseases. Two different diagnoses. But the same root cause. And that root cause, as I have come to understand through years of research, is insulin resistance.

When I first wrote about this in *The Fibre First Diet*, I knew the statistics. Insulin resistance multiplies the risk of Alzheimer's by five times. Five times. Not 5%. Five times. That makes it one of the most significant modifiable risk factors for a disease that is currently destroying millions of families across the world.

• • •

Type 3 Diabetes

In many medical and research circles, Alzheimer's disease is now being called type 3 diabetes. That is not a metaphor. It is not a shorthand. It is a clinical description of what is actually happening inside the brain. Personally, I would prefer to call it "type 2 diabetes of the brain", because that is exactly what it is. The same insulin resistance, the same mechanism, just in a different organ.

Your brain is the most energy-hungry organ in your body. It makes up roughly 2% of your body weight, but it consumes around 20% of your energy. It is absolutely dependent on a reliable fuel supply, and under normal conditions, much of that fuel comes from glucose.

But here is the critical detail. Glucose cannot just walk into a brain cell. It needs insulin to help it get there. Insulin plays a vital role in brain glucose metabolism and in the signalling between neurons. Without proper insulin function, the brain's ability to access glucose is compromised. Think back to what Ben told us earlier, in a petri dish you can have cells sitting in a sea of glucose, but without insulin they cannot take it in. The neurons could be surrounded by fuel and still starving.

Now think about what happens when you have been running chronically elevated insulin for ten, twenty, thirty years. The same thing that happens in your muscles, your fat and your liver can happen in your brain. The brain's cells become insulin resistant. They stop responding properly to insulin's signal.

The result is devastating, and it is deeply counterintuitive. As just mentioned, the brain can be swimming in glucose. There can be plenty of sugar in the blood, plenty circulating around the neurons. But the neurons cannot access it. Imagine standing in front of a locked pantry, starving, while you can see the shelves are full of food through the glass door. The food is right there. You just cannot get to it. That is what is happening to the neurons in an Alzheimer's brain. They are energy-starved in the midst of plenty.

And when neurons are starved of energy, they start to malfunction. They lose the ability to form new connections. They struggle to maintain existing ones. Memory falters. Cognitive function declines. And eventually, the neurons begin to die.

• • •

When the Door to the Brain Locks and Then Breaks

One of the things I have always tried to do when researching any health subject is read as widely as possible, even when the science gets uncomfortable or seems to challenge what I think I know. So, when Dr Georgia Ede published her book *Change Your Diet, Change Your Mind*, I picked it up straight away. And when I later started working with Isabella, I thought at first that what she was now explaining to me about the cause of Alzheimer's conflicted with what Dr Ede had written.

To understand what they were both describing, you need to know a little about the *blood-brain barrier*. Your brain is the most protected organ in your body. It sits behind a tightly sealed wall of cells called the blood-brain barrier, or BBB, which controls what gets in and what stays out. Imagine the finest mesh filter you have ever seen, stretched across every blood vessel that feeds the brain. The cells that form this barrier are packed together so tightly that there are no gaps between them. Most things in your blood cannot cross it. Toxins, bacteria, large molecules, they are all blocked. Only specific substances with their own dedicated transport vehicles are allowed through. Glucose gets a pass, carried across by GLUT1 transporters. Ketones get through via

MCT transporters. Oxygen diffuses across freely. But almost everything else is turned away at the door.

Insulin is one of those substances. It does not simply drift into the brain. It needs specialised insulin receptors on the barrier wall to carry it across, a process scientists call receptor-mediated transcytosis. In a healthy person, this system works perfectly. Insulin binds to the receptor on the blood side of the barrier, is pulled through the cell in a tiny package, and released on the brain side, where it plays a vital role in helping neurons take in glucose, in memory formation, and in the signalling between brain cells.

And the brain needs that glucose desperately. Unlike your muscles and your liver, which can store glucose as glycogen and draw on it later, your brain has no energy reserves at all. It consumes roughly 20% of your entire energy supply, every minute of every day, and it needs a constant, uninterrupted flow of fuel to do so. When that flow is disrupted, even briefly, the consequences are immediate.

Now think about what happens when the transporters at the blood-brain barrier become insulin resistant. They stop responding properly. Less insulin gets shuttled across. And without insulin on the other side of the barrier, the brain cells cannot access the glucose that is flowing right past them. Dr Ede describes exactly this process in her book, and she also spoke about this on stage at one of our conferences, emphasising that metabolic health and insulin control are central to protecting memory.

At first, that sounded like the opposite of what Isabella was describing. Isabella's research shows that over time, chronically high insulin does not just impair the transporters. It damages the blood-brain barrier itself. The tightly sealed wall that is supposed to protect your brain starts to break down. When that happens, insulin is no longer carefully shuttled across in controlled amounts. It floods through in waves, far more than the brain was ever designed to receive.

And just like the cells in your muscles and your liver, the neurons respond to this constant bombardment by becoming insulin resistant. They stop listening. So now you have brain cells that are surrounded by insulin but can no longer respond to it, which means they can no longer take in the glucose they need to function. The fuel is there. The signal is there. But the connection between the two is broken.

The more I sat with these two different pathologies, the more I realised both experts are describing different stages of the same process. In the early stage, the transporters fail, starving the brain of insulin and therefore glucose. The door locks. Later, the barrier itself breaks down, letting in abnormally high levels of insulin and inflammation that push neurons into full-blown insulin resistance. And in both stages, the story circles back to the same place: insulin resistance and the metabolic chaos it creates.

But if insulin struggles to cross a damaged blood-brain barrier, what about the other nutrients your brain desperately needs? There is an important distinction here. When we talk about insulin struggling to cross the blood-brain barrier, we are talking about a large peptide hormone that relies on its own receptor-mediated transport system. When that system breaks down under insulin resistance, insulin can no longer get through efficiently, and the brain starts to starve.

Omega-3 fatty acids, specifically DHA, have a different dedicated transport system, a protein called Mfsd2a that sits on the blood-brain barrier and actively pulls DHA across. The brain needs DHA. It is one of the primary building blocks of neuronal membranes. Crucially, DHA transport does not depend on insulin signalling, so it does not break down in the same way when insulin resistance develops.

This supports the bigger picture. A brain with good omega-3 intake has healthier cell membranes, less inflammation, and a better-functioning blood-brain barrier. When omega-3 is low, inflammation rises, the barrier degrades, insulin transport fails, and you are back on the road to metabolic damage in the brain. Omega-3 does not contradict the insulin story. It reinforces it.

The blood-brain barrier has dedicated transport systems for more than just insulin and DHA. Each B vitamin has its own carrier proteins that shuttle it across. Fat-soluble vitamins like D, E, and K have a natural advantage because the barrier itself is made of lipid membranes. Minerals like zinc, iron, and magnesium each have their own transporters too. The brain is the most energy-hungry organ in your body, and it has built customs checkpoints for everything it needs. The question is not whether these nutrients can get across. The question is whether those transport systems are working properly. And this is where it circles back to insulin. Chronic inflammation and metabolic dysfunction damage the blood-brain barrier itself, which disrupts all of these transport systems, not just the one for insulin. A well-nourished brain has a healthier barrier. A healthier barrier lets everything through that should get through. It all starts with the same thing.

• • •

The Brain's Night Shift

The damage does not only happen during the day. In fact, some of the most important damage can happen at night, while you sleep. And once again, chronically elevated insulin is a key player.

We talked in the cancer chapter about *melatonin*, the sleep hormone, and how it can be suppressed when insulin is chronically high. Melatonin does much more than help you fall asleep. It is one of the most powerful antioxidants in the body and plays a critical role in protecting the brain during sleep.

While you sleep, your brain runs its housekeeping programmes. It clears out waste products, repairs damaged neurons, and consolidates memories. Melatonin supports all of this. As we mentioned earlier, melatonin helps keep *HIF-1α low*, which allows brain cells to burn glucose more cleanly in their mitochondria, rather than shifting toward the more wasteful glycolysis pathway.

When melatonin production is suppressed by chronically high insulin, two things can happen. First, the brain's nighttime repair and clearance systems run less efficiently. Waste products accumulate, and damaged cells are not cleared as effectively. This impairment is one of the mechanisms by which the amyloid plaques and tau tangles characteristic of Alzheimer's disease are allowed to build up. The rubbish collectors have been sent home.

Second, without melatonin to help keep HIF-1α and related pathways in check, glucose metabolism in parts of the brain can shift toward a more inefficient, fermentation-like pattern. Mitochondria start producing excessive reactive oxygen species, which cause further damage to neurons that are already struggling to get enough energy.

So, the brain is left simultaneously starving for fuel, drowning in waste products, and being damaged by its own stressed energy-production systems. And one of the upstream drivers of this trouble is insulin that has been too high for too long.

• • •

The Bone-Brain Connection

This is where Isabella shared something that genuinely astonished me. It is one of those pieces of science that, when you first hear it, sounds like it cannot possibly be true. Yet it is. And it may be one of the most important discoveries in brain health in recent decades.

There is a protein hormone called *osteocalcin.* Most people have never heard of it. But as Isabella explained:

"Osteocalcin is a protein hormone. It is made by your bone cells inside your bones. It is sending messages to your pancreas and it is telling your pancreas how much insulin to make and how much glucagon to make. It triggers GLP-1 receptors as well."

So here is a hormone made by your bones that is talking to your pancreas, regulating your insulin production, and activating the very GLP-1 receptors that weight loss injections are designed to target. But that is not the extraordinary part.

The extraordinary part is what happens in the brain. Osteocalcin crosses the blood-brain barrier. Once inside the brain, it does something that no drug on the market can reliably do. As Isabella put it:

"Osteocalcin stimulates neurogenesis in the hippocampus. IQ, brain power, very, very important."

Neurogenesis. The creation of new brain cells. In the hippocampus, the part of the brain most associated with memory and learning. The very part of the brain that Alzheimer's attacks first. Your bones are making a hormone that creates new brain cells. Let that sink in for a moment.

But osteocalcin production requires low insulin. When insulin is chronically elevated, osteocalcin is suppressed. The signal from your bones to your brain gets weaker. Fewer new brain cells are created. The hippocampus loses its ability to regenerate. And the decline towards dementia accelerates.

Osteocalcin also triggers the production of serotonin and dopamine, two of the brain's most important signalling molecules. Serotonin regulates mood, sleep, and appetite. Dopamine drives motivation, pleasure, and reward. When osteocalcin drops because insulin is high, serotonin and dopamine production both fall. This is one of the reasons why depression, anxiety, and low motivation are so common in people with metabolic dysfunction. It is not just a psychological problem. It is a biochemical one, rooted in the same hormonal imbalance that drives Alzheimer's.

• • •

The Methylation Problem

There is another pathway by which insulin can damage the brain, and it runs through something called the *methylation* system. I'm going to keep this as simple as possible, because the biochemistry gets complex, but the principle is straightforward.

Methylation is one of your body's most important chemical processes. In simple terms, it is your body's way of switching genes on and off, and of keeping your cells running cleanly. Every second, billions of tiny chemical tags called methyl groups are being attached to your DNA, your proteins, and your neurotransmitters. These tags control everything from DNA repair to detoxification to the production of the brain chemicals that regulate your mood. For the system to work, your body needs a steady supply of three key nutrients: vitamin B12, folate, and a substance called betaine, which your body makes from choline, a nutrient found in eggs, liver, and fish.

Chronically elevated insulin reduces stomach acid and alters nutrient metabolism, impairing the methylation system in two ways. First, reduced stomach acid limits the absorption of B12 from food, so less of this vital methylation nutrient reaches the bloodstream. Second, high insulin impairs your body's ability to convert choline into betaine, another essential methylation nutrient.

When the methylation system fails, a toxic amino acid called homocysteine builds up in the blood. Elevated homocysteine is one of the most well-established risk factors for Alzheimer's disease. It damages blood vessels in the brain, promotes inflammation, and directly harms neurons. It has been linked to brain shrinkage, cognitive decline, and the progression from mild memory problems to full dementia.

And the root cause of the elevated homocysteine? Damaged methylation. Caused by chronically elevated insulin. The trail leads back to the same place it always does. The insulin problem.

• • •

The Metabolism-Neurology Connection

For decades, medicine treated metabolic diseases and neurological diseases as completely separate fields. Diabetes was the endocrinologist's problem. Alzheimer's was the neurologist's problem. The two departments rarely spoke to each other. As I recently described it to a journalist:

"There used to be a dualism, where the medical community believed diseases only below the neck to be metabolically driven, but above the neck to be neurological. But now we're beginning to realise that a lot of neurological issues actually relate to metabolism too."

That wall between metabolism and neurology is finally starting to crumble. Researchers are now recognising that Alzheimer's, Parkinson's, depression, anxiety, and even conditions like ADHD all have metabolic components. They all involve, to varying degrees, mitochondrial dysfunction, insulin signalling problems, and the suppression of the very hormones and molecules that keep the brain healthy: osteocalcin, melatonin, serotonin, and dopamine.

This is not to say that every case of Alzheimer's is caused by insulin resistance. Genetics play a role. The APOE4 gene, which increases Alzheimer's risk, is well documented, and I carry it. But even here, the picture is more nuanced than it first appears. Research suggests that the APOE4 gene is not as harmful as previously thought if insulin is kept low and ketosis is maintained. In other words, even if you have the genetic predisposition, the metabolic environment determines whether that gene expresses itself as disease. My gun is loaded, but it is insulin that might pull the trigger.

• • •

The Alternative Fuel

There is a piece of hope in all of this, and it is important.

The brain does not have to run on glucose. It can run, very efficiently, on ketones. In fact, there is growing evidence that ketones may not just be an alternative fuel for the brain. They may be its preferred one.

Ben Bikman put this to rest emphatically describing how, even after a relatively short fast of around 24 hours, blood ketone levels might reach roughly one mmol/L, while blood glucose sits at around five mmol/L, five times higher. And yet, even in that scenario, the brain has already switched to drawing the majority of its energy from ketones. As Ben put it:

"Do not tell me the brain prefers glucose when glucose is five times more available and the brain is still choosing ketones.

The moment ketones hit the bloodstream, the brain starts pulling them in."

When insulin is low and the body is burning fat, the liver produces ketones. These ketones cross the blood-brain barrier easily and provide energy directly to neurons, bypassing the broken transporters entirely. It is like finding a back door into that locked pantry. The transporters needed to unlock glucose may be dysfunctional, but the ketone transporters still work perfectly well.

This is why some of the most promising research into Alzheimer's prevention and early-stage treatment involves ketogenic diets, intermittent fasting, and even supplemental ketones. When you give the brain an alternative fuel source, one that does not depend on insulin signalling to get in, the neurons can access the energy they need. Cognitive function stabilises. In some cases, it improves.

I have experienced this firsthand. When I ran four marathons in five days, completely fasted as an experiment with a bunch of my doctor friends, something extraordinary happened. As my ketone levels increased, dreams became more vivid than anything I had ever experienced. During the day, I saw colours I had never noticed before. Sounds were sharper, clearer, more alive. My brain was not shutting down from lack of food. It was waking up. I wasn't the only one this happened to, all nine of us partaking in the experiment had similar experiences.

Two years later in a follow-up experiment, I rode five hundred miles from Glasgow to Bristol on my pushbike. Double Gold Medal Olympian James Cracknell rode with me. Because he had suffered a serious brain injury falling off his bike exactly ten years to the day before we set off, his PR team were nervous. They felt it was too dangerous, even foolish, to cycle such a long way without food and advised him not to do it. The reality was the exact opposite. Our brains were more alert without food than they had ever been with it. When you strip away the constant glucose bombardment and let the brain run on ketones, it does not suffer. It thrives.

Even supplementing with ketones, without a full dietary change, has shown benefits. This is not a cure for established Alzheimer's. I am not claiming that. But it is evidence that the brain's energy crisis can be at least partially addressed by changing what fuel is available.

In my book *The Fibre First Diet*, I told the story of Dr Mary Newport, a physician and acclaimed author of five books on Alzheimer's, and what happened when she changed her husband Steve's diet. Steve had Alzheimer's and was deteriorating. He could not draw a clock face, one of the standard cognitive tests used to assess the disease. Mary began incorporating coconut oil enriched with a compound called C8 into his meals, which shifted his brain into a ketogenic state, giving his neurons an alternative fuel that did not depend on the broken insulin signalling. Within fourteen days, his clock drawings improved. By thirty-seven days, he drew a recognisable clock with clarity and ease. His brain had not healed. But it had found fuel it could actually use.

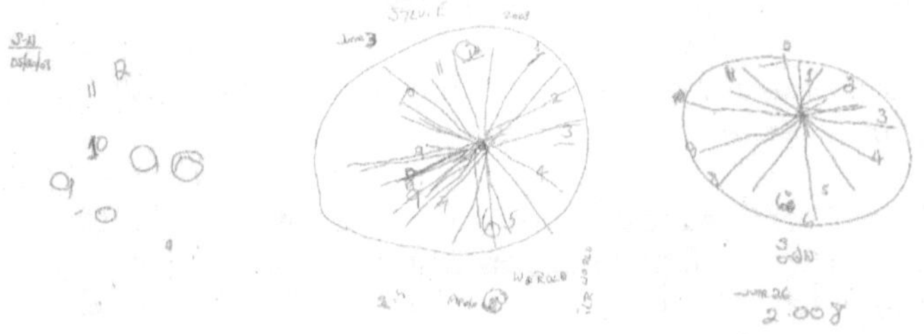

1 day before coconut oil | 14 days after starting coconut oil | 37 days after starting coconut oil

I share this not as a miracle story, but as evidence. The science in this chapter is not theoretical. It is already changing lives. And if a brain as damaged as Steve Newport's could respond to a simple change in fuel, imagine what protecting your insulin sensitivity now, before any damage is done, could mean for your future.

• • •

It Is Not Just Alzheimer's

What we have discussed so far about insulin resistance starving the brain of energy does not only apply to Alzheimer's. The same metabolic dysfunction is showing up across a whole range of neurological and mental health conditions. As Dr Christopher Palmer explained to me during our meeting in London, mental illnesses are fundamentally metabolic disorders of the brain. Depression, anxiety, schizophrenia, bipolar disorder, ADHD, migraines, epilepsy. All rising at alarming rates. All increasingly being linked to the same underlying problem: the brain is not getting the fuel it needs.

Epilepsy is perhaps the most established example. In the UK alone, around 600,000 people live with the condition, and for roughly 30% of them, medications simply do not work. What most people do not realise is that for over a hundred years, the ketogenic diet has been used to treat those with epilepsy. The approach was developed in 1923 by Dr Russell Wilder at the Mayo Clinic, and it worked remarkably well, significantly reducing seizures in over half of patients.

Then pharmaceutical anticonvulsants arrived in the 1940s and the diet was quietly forgotten. It took a father's desperation to bring it back. In 1993, Jim Abrahams took his son Charlie, who was suffering from severe drug-resistant epilepsy, to Johns Hopkins University. Charlie was put on a ketogenic diet and his seizures virtually disappeared. Jim went on to write a screenplay about the experience, *First Do No Harm*, starring Meryl Streep, and the resulting publicity helped relaunch interest in ketogenic therapy worldwide. The science behind it is elegant: by switching the brain's fuel source from glucose to ketones, you change its electrical dynamics. The storms that cause seizures begin to quieten.

Then there is bipolar disorder, and the story of Matt Baszucki is one of the most powerful I have come across. Matt was diagnosed at 19. Over the years that followed, he tried 29 different medications and saw 40 different doctors. Nothing worked. His condition was classified as treatment-resistant, which in medical language meant the pharmaceutical industry had given up. His parents, Jan and David Baszucki, refused to accept that. They found Dr Christopher Palmer, who put Matt on a ketogenic diet starting on the 4th of January 2021. The results were remarkable. Matt's mood stabilised. His mental clarity improved. Even his psychiatrist, who had been sceptical, admitted the transformation was extraordinary. Today, Matt works a full-time job and has spoken publicly about his recovery. His story was not fixed by a new drug. It was fixed by food.

What ties all of this together is the same principle we keep returning to. When brain cells become insulin resistant, they lose access to glucose. They start to malfunction. Whether that malfunction shows up as memory loss, seizures, mood instability, or depression depends on which part of the brain is affected. But the root cause is the same. And the solution, restoring the brain's energy supply through ketones, keeps proving itself across conditions that mainstream medicine still treats as entirely separate diseases.

• • •

Why This Matters to Me

I watched my mum lose herself. There is no other way to describe it. Alzheimer's does not just steal your memory. It steals your personality, your relationships, your dignity, and eventually your life. It is one of the cruellest diseases I have ever witnessed.

My dad, eating the same meals at the same table for the same seventy years, developed type 2 diabetes instead. Different branch of the same tree. The same trunk, the same root. Insulin resistance.

I cannot go back and change what happened to my parents. But I can make sure that other people understand what I did not understand in time. That Alzheimer's is not random. That in many cases, it is the end point of decades of metabolic damage. That the same dietary patterns that drive obesity and diabetes also starve the brain of energy, suppress the hormones that create new brain cells, disable the nighttime repair systems, and poison the methylation pathways that keep neurons healthy.

And I can tell you, with the confidence that comes from seeing the science laid out in front of me by one of the most brilliant biochemists I have ever met, that managing your insulin is the single most powerful thing you can do to protect your brain.

Not a pill. Not a scan. Not a diagnosis you receive when it is already too late. A choice you make at every meal, starting today.

CHAPTER SIX

How Insulin Causes Heart Disease

• • •

Although recent reports now suggest that Alzheimer's and dementia have overtaken it as the number one cause of premature death in the UK, other research still places cardiovascular disease slightly ahead. Either way, it has held that title for decades. And for decades, we have been told the same story about why. Too much *cholesterol* in the blood. Too much saturated fat in the diet. Too much use of the salt shaker.

That story is wrong. Not entirely wrong, but wrong in the way that matters most. Wrong about the root cause. Wrong about what to measure. And wrong about what to do about it.

The real story, the one that the evidence increasingly supports, is that heart disease is primarily a disease of insulin. And once you understand why, the standard dietary advice that we have been given for the last fifty years starts to look not just misguided, but actively dangerous.

• • •

The Cholesterol Misdirection

Let me start with *cholesterol*, because it is the elephant in the room and we need to deal with it head-on.

For half a century, we have been told that *LDL cholesterol*, the so-called bad cholesterol, is the primary driver of heart disease. That it clogs your arteries. That you need to get it as low as possible. That if your number is above a certain threshold, you should be on a statin for the rest of your life.

I am not going to tell you that cholesterol has nothing to do with heart disease. That would be an oversimplification. But I am going to tell you something that may surprise you, and it comes from studying multiple pieces of research and interpreting them correctly.

In hazard ratio studies, which measure how well different markers predict cardiovascular death, *hyperinsulinaemia* (too much insulin in the blood) is a stronger predictor than LDL cholesterol. Let me say that again. If you want to know who is most likely to have a heart attack, measuring their insulin is more useful than measuring their cholesterol.

That does not mean cholesterol is irrelevant. But it does mean that we have spent fifty years fixated on the wrong number. We have been measuring cholesterol while ignoring insulin, and the result has been an epidemic of heart disease that no amount of statins has been able to reverse.

I do not want to sound cynical, and that is not what this book is about. But it is worth asking the question: why has medicine focused so heavily on cholesterol while largely ignoring insulin? Well, if you blame elevated cholesterol, you can sell a drug to bring it down. Statins are one of the most prescribed medications on the planet. But if you blame elevated insulin, the solution is not a pill. It is moving your food choices away from the products made by big food corporations and towards the food grown by your local farmer. That is not good for profit. Not for the pharmaceutical industry, and not for the processed food industry. Two of the largest commercial sectors in the world, both with a vested interest in making sure the conversation stays exactly where it is.

• • •

What LDL Actually Does

Here is something that most people do not know, because the standard cholesterol narrative never mentions it. LDL particles are not just lumps of fat floating around your blood looking for arteries to block. They are delivery vehicles.

LDL particles carry cholesterol, yes. But they also carry essential fatty acids, fat-soluble vitamins A, D, E, and K, and a substance called taurine, which is critical for mitochondrial function. Their job is to transport these vital nutrients to the cells that need them. Cholesterol itself is essential for the health of every cell membrane in your body. Without it, your cells literally cannot function.

When you take a statin and drive LDL down as low as possible, you are not just reducing cholesterol. You are reducing the delivery of essential nutrients to your cells. This is one of the reasons why, counterintuitively, research has shown that people with higher cholesterol levels tend to have better cancer prognoses, and people with very low cholesterol tend to have worse outcomes. The cells are nutrient-depleted. They are less able to resist disease.

None of this means you should ignore dangerously high cholesterol. But it does mean that the simplistic narrative of LDL equals bad is not telling you the full story. And the part of the story that is missing? Insulin.

Check this out. A Swedish population study published in the journal GeroScience in 2023, which Ben Bikman first brought to my attention, looked at the blood biomarkers of people who survived beyond 100. Three variables stood out above all others: good glucose control, low uric acid, and high total cholesterol.

That last one should stop you in your tracks. The people who lived the longest did not have the lowest cholesterol. They had higher cholesterol than the general population. Their cholesterol was left alone to do what it is supposed to do: build cell membranes, construct hormones, fuel mitochondria, and fight infections.

What they did have was low, stable blood sugar, which means their insulin was working properly. The longest-lived people in Sweden were simply metabolically healthy. As Ben said to me:

"We could be doing the perfectly wrong thing to help people live longer."

If the medical establishment is spending billions lowering a molecule the body needs, while ignoring the hormone that is actually driving the damage, you have to ask yourself: who benefits from that?

• • •

How Insulin Damages Your Arteries

So, if cholesterol is not the primary villain, what is actually causing heart disease? The answer involves several mechanisms, all of them driven by chronically elevated insulin. Let me walk you through them one at a time.

Endothelial damage. The inside of every artery in your body is lined with a thin layer of cells called the endothelium. Think of it as the wallpaper inside your blood vessels. When it is smooth and healthy, blood flows freely. When it is damaged, rough patches form, and that is where problems begin. Chronically elevated insulin directly damages the endothelium. It causes chronic low-level inflammation in the artery walls, and it triggers the growth of cells in the arterial lining. These are the same growth-promoting pathways we discussed in the cancer chapter. VEGF, the growth factor that builds blood vessels for tumours, also promotes unhealthy growth in arterial walls. And insulin drives VEGF production.

Blood viscosity. This is a mechanism that Isabella explained to me, and it changed how I think about blood pressure. When your blood glucose is high, your blood literally becomes thicker. More viscous. Your kidneys detect this increased viscosity and respond by retaining water to dilute the blood. That water retention raises your blood volume, which raises your blood pressure.

For decades, we have been told that salt causes high blood pressure. Cut down on salt, your doctor says, and your blood pressure will drop. But the research increasingly suggests that in many people, it is not the salt that is causing the water retention. It is the glucose. The kidneys are retaining water to dilute thick, sugary blood, not salty blood. Salt has been blamed for a problem that glucose is causing.

This does not mean that extreme salt intake is harmless. But it does mean that millions of people are cutting salt while continuing to eat the carbohydrates that are actually driving their blood pressure up.

There is another mechanism at work too. Chronically elevated insulin stimulates the production of *aldosterone*, a hormone made by your adrenal glands that tells your kidneys to retain sodium. Where sodium goes, water follows. So, insulin is raising your blood pressure from two directions at once: thickening the blood with glucose, and telling the kidneys to hold onto more fluid through aldosterone. Your doctor prescribes a pill to lower blood pressure. But the insulin that is driving the aldosterone that is raising the blood pressure goes unmeasured and untreated.

The hormone disruption. Excess insulin triggers the production of an enzyme called *aromatase*. Aromatase converts testosterone into oestrogen. In men, this means that chronically high insulin is effectively feminising their hormonal profile. Testosterone drops. Oestrogen rises. And this hormonal imbalance has direct effects on cardiovascular function. Testosterone is protective for the heart and blood vessels. When it falls and oestrogen rises inappropriately, vascular dysfunction follows.

This is one of the reasons why men are at their highest risk of stroke and heart attack around age fifty-five. By that point, decades of elevated insulin have depleted their testosterone and elevated their oestrogen through the aromatase pathway. The protective hormonal balance has been tipped.

Mitochondrial damage and HIF-1α. We covered HIF-1α in the cancer chapter, but its effects are not limited to tumours. When HIF-1α is chronically elevated in heart tissue, which happens when insulin is too high and melatonin production is suppressed, it can actually kill heart cells. Not just damage them. Kill them. This is direct, insulin-driven destruction of the heart muscle itself.

• • •

Why Women Are Protected, Until They Are Not

There is an interesting gender difference in heart disease that makes more sense once you understand insulin.

Before menopause, women are far less likely to suffer heart attacks and strokes than men of the same age. This has always been put down to oestrogen. And oestrogen does play a role. But there are two other protections that rarely get mentioned.

The first is SHBG. Younger women naturally have higher levels of it. As we saw in the cancer chapter, SHBG binds to hormones and controls how they signal to cells. When SHBG is high, the damaging effects of excess insulin are kept in check. It acts as a buffer.

The second is iron. Women lose iron every month through menstruation. That sounds like a disadvantage, but it turns out to be protective. Excess iron drives insulin resistance. The monthly loss keeps iron levels lower, giving women a degree of metabolic protection that men simply do not have.

After menopause, both of these disappear. SHBG drops as insulin resistance builds over the years. The monthly iron loss stops. And almost overnight, women's heart disease risk climbs sharply, eventually matching and sometimes exceeding men's.

This is usually described as women losing the protection of oestrogen. But it would be more accurate to say they lose the mechanisms that were shielding them from the damage insulin had been doing all along. The insulin was always there. The damage was always accumulating. The shield just finally came down.

• • •

The ACCORD Trial: When More Insulin Made Things Worse

If you need any further evidence that insulin, not glucose, is the real problem, consider the ACCORD trial.

ACCORD was one of the largest clinical trials ever conducted on type 2 diabetes. Over ten thousand participants. The question was simple: if we aggressively lower blood sugar in diabetics, using intensive insulin therapy, will they have fewer heart attacks and live longer?

The participants were split into two groups. One group received moderate insulin therapy, targeting an *HbA1c* of 7.1 to 7.9%. The other group received intensive insulin therapy, targeting an HbA1c below 6%. Lower blood sugar. Tighter control. The standard medical assumption was that the intensive group would do much better.

They did not. The intensive insulin group had approximately twenty-six more deaths than the moderate group. The trial was stopped early because people in the intensive group were dying faster.

Think about that. The group that received *more insulin* and achieved *lower blood sugar* had *worse outcomes*. Yes, they achieved lower blood sugar, but they died more. Not less. More.

This result baffled the medical establishment, but it makes perfect sense once you understand that insulin itself is the problem. Forcing blood sugar down by flooding the body with even more insulin does not make you healthier. It makes you sicker. You are treating the symptom (high glucose) by amplifying the cause (high insulin). It is like trying to put out a fire by pouring petrol on it, then celebrating because the temperature gauge briefly dropped.

• • •

The Doctor Who Got It Right

In *The Fibre First Diet*, I wrote about Dr Joseph Kraft, a pathologist who spent decades studying the relationship between insulin and cardiovascular disease. His conclusion was as blunt as it was profound. He said that people with cardiovascular disease who have not been identified as having diabetes, meaning insulin resistance, are simply undiagnosed.

In other words, if you have heart disease, you almost certainly have insulin resistance. You just have not been tested for it. Because nobody is testing for it. They are testing your cholesterol. They are testing your blood pressure. They are prescribing statins and blood pressure medication. But they are not measuring the one thing that is driving the whole process.

This is not a fringe opinion. The evidence is there. Hyperinsulinaemia is the strongest predictor of cardiovascular morbidity and mortality. Stronger than LDL. Stronger than blood pressure. Stronger than any of the markers that your GP is currently checking.

• • •

The Real Solution

If heart disease is primarily driven by insulin, then the solution is not more drugs. It is not lower cholesterol targets or stricter blood pressure medication. It is addressing the insulin.

And the most powerful way to address your insulin is through what you eat. Reduce the sugar and carbohydrates that are constantly spiking your insulin. Stop the endless cycle of glucose bombardment that is thickening your blood, inflaming your arteries, disrupting your hormones, and damaging your heart cells.

I realise that this contradicts almost everything you have been told. For fifty years, the dietary advice for preventing heart disease has been: cut the fat, eat more whole grains, reduce your cholesterol. But that advice has coincided with an explosion in heart disease, obesity, and type 2 diabetes. The advice is not working. And the reason it is not working is that it has been targeting the wrong thing.

Heart disease is not primarily a fat problem. It is not primarily a cholesterol problem. It is not primarily a salt problem. At its root, for millions of people, it is an insulin problem. And insulin is something you can manage, starting with your very next meal.

As I have said before, this is not medical advice. If you are on medication for your heart, do not stop taking it based on anything I have written. But do ask questions. Ask your GP about your insulin levels. Ask why they have never been measured. Ask whether there is a conversation to be had about diet alongside your medication. You deserve to understand the full picture, not just the part that fits neatly into a prescription.

CHAPTER SEVEN

The Diabetes & Liver Trap

. . .

Most health professionals consider type 2 diabetes to be a chronic, progressive and irreversible disease. A one-way street. A life sentence with no possibility of parole. The disease continually gets worse until you eventually require insulin injections. You are given medication to manage it and told to accept that this is your reality now.

That is a lie. It is one of the most damaging lies in modern medicine. And in this chapter, I am going to explain why.

Type 2 diabetes is, in the overwhelming majority of cases, reversible. Not manageable. Not treatable. Reversible. People are doing it every day, often within weeks, by addressing the one thing that the standard treatment ignores: the insulin.

My good friend Dr David Unwin, who sits on our advisory panel at Clubwell, has been proving this in his NHS practice for years. He has helped hundreds of patients put their type 2 diabetes into remission through dietary changes alone, saving the NHS a fortune in medication costs in the process. He once sent the NHS a cheque for £40,000 — for unused diabetes drugs! David has proven that this works, not in a laboratory, not in theory, but in a real GP surgery with real patients.

It is one of my biggest personal ambitions to help as many people as possible discover this truth and reverse their diabetes. Not manage it. Reverse it. Because nobody should have to live with a disease that, for most people, does not have to exist.

The Wrong Treatment for the Right Disease

To understand why the standard treatment for type 2 diabetes is so badly flawed, you need to understand what the disease actually is. And what it actually is, as we have discussed throughout this book, is the insulin, or more correctly, insulin resistance.

For those diagnosed with type 2 diabetes, their cells have been bombarded with insulin for so long that they have stopped responding to it. Their blood sugar rises because insulin can no longer push glucose into the cells efficiently. So, their doctor measures their blood sugar, sees that it is too high, and prescribes a medication to bring it down. That medication might be metformin. It might be a sulfonylurea. And eventually, in many cases, it is insulin injections.

Think about that for a moment. Their body has too much insulin. Their cells have stopped responding to it because there is too much of it. And the medical response is to give them more of it.

The blood sugar does come down. Their *HbA1c* looks better on paper. Their doctor tells them the medication is working. But the diabetes has not improved. It has got worse. Because the underlying problem, the excess insulin, has been amplified, not addressed.

Dr Jason Fung, one of the world's leading experts on diabetes reversal, puts it starkly:

"The blood glucose got better with insulin, but the diabetes got worse. The medication only hid the blood glucose by cramming it into the already engorged cells. The diabetes looks better, but it is worse."

It is like treating a flooding house by buying bigger buckets. The water level in the hallway goes down temporarily. The house looks drier. But the pipe is still burst, and the water is still coming in faster than you can bail it out. Sooner or later, you run out of buckets.

• • •

The Silent Decades

One of the most frightening aspects of type 2 diabetes is how long it can develop without being detected. My dad is the perfect example. For years he battled gout, an unwelcome companion that had been shadowing him for as long as I can remember. Then came high blood pressure. Then came the discreet conversations we had about Viagra. Each one was a separate visit to his GP, treated as a separate problem, a separate prescription. Nobody joined the dots. It was not until his late seventies that he was finally diagnosed with type 2 diabetes. But if you look at my *Tree of Afflictions* diagram, every single one of those conditions is a branch on the same tree. They are all expressions of insulin resistance. The gout, the blood pressure, the erectile dysfunction, the diabetes. They were never separate problems. They were warning flares, fired one after another over decades, and every single one was missed.

The standard diagnostic test is HbA1c, which measures your average blood sugar over the previous three months. If it comes back normal, you are told you are fine. But as we have discussed in earlier chapters, you can have normal blood sugar for ten, fifteen, even twenty years while your insulin is dangerously elevated. The sugar looks normal because the insulin is working overtime to keep it down. It is only when either the pancreas finally becomes exhausted, the beta cells that produce insulin start to burn out, or the cells of the body become extremely insulin resistant that blood sugar begins to rise and you get your diagnosis.

By that point, the damage has been accumulating silently for decades. The excess insulin has already been feeding cancer cells, damaging your brain, inflaming your arteries, and corrupting your liver. The diabetes diagnosis is not the beginning of the disease. It is the end of a long process of metabolic destruction that nobody was monitoring.

This is why I keep returning to the same point throughout this book. We are measuring the wrong thing. HbA1c tells you what your blood sugar has been doing. It tells you nothing about what your insulin has been doing. And it is the insulin that drives the damage.

• • •

What Diabetes Does to the Body

If you have type 2 diabetes, or you know someone who does, this next section may be difficult to read. But I believe you need to understand the full picture, because understanding it is the first step towards doing something about it.

When blood sugar is consistently elevated over years and decades, it damages every organ in the body. There is no tissue that is spared. The eyes deteriorate to such a state that diabetes is the leading cause of blindness among working-age adults in the UK.

The kidneys fail, leading to dialysis. The heart weakens, leading to heart attacks and heart failure. The brain degenerates, accelerating the path towards Alzheimer's. The liver fills with fat, leading to fatty liver disease and eventually cirrhosis.

The nerves are destroyed, causing neuropathy, that painful tingling and numbness that starts in the feet and works its way up. And the circulation in the extremities becomes so poor that tissue dies. In the UK, over 176 leg, toe, or foot amputations are performed every single week on people with type 2 diabetes. Every week. Diabetes is now the number one cause for amputations in the UK, not accidents.

The following is probably the most frightening statistic in this book, so I want you to read it slowly.

Research led by Dr Adrian Heald, a consultant diabetologist in the UK, analysed data from the National Diabetes Audit covering millions of patients. His findings were stark. If your HbA1c consistently sits above 58 mmol/mol, you are looking at losing roughly one third of your remaining lifespan. Let me put that another way. For every year you live with poorly controlled diabetes, you lose one hundred days. Not one hundred hours. One hundred days. Gone. Over a million people in the UK are currently in that category, most of them being managed with medication while the insulin driving their condition goes unmeasured.

These are not abstract statistics. These are people's parents, partners, children, and friends. And the tragedy is that for most of them, this disease did not have to happen.

• • •

The Obesity Connection

Type 2 diabetes and obesity are so closely linked that they are sometimes referred to together as diabesity. But the relationship between the two is widely misunderstood.

The conventional view is that being overweight causes diabetes. Lose weight, and your diabetes will improve. That is partly true, but it misses the underlying mechanism. It is not the fat itself that causes the diabetes. It's the insulin.

Remember what Ben Bikman showed me in his laboratory. Fat cells sitting in a petri dish, surrounded by sugar, surrounded by energy, surrounded by calories, will not grow. They cannot take up the energy. But add a dash of insulin, and they soak it up like a sponge. Insulin is the gatekeeper. Without it, fat cells cannot store fat, no matter how many calories are available.

This is why calorie counting alone so often fails to reverse diabetes. You can cut your calories to starvation levels, and if your insulin remains high, your body will continue to store fat. It will slow your metabolism to compensate for the reduced intake. It will make you hungrier, more tired, and more miserable. But it will not let go of the fat, because insulin is still giving the order to hold on to it.

The real driver of both obesity and type 2 diabetes is not calories. It is elevated insulin. And elevated insulin is driven by what you eat, specifically by the volume of carbohydrates that are constantly spiking your blood sugar, constantly demanding an insulin response, and constantly overwhelming a system that was never designed to handle this level of load.

And the genetics argument? It does not hold up either. Only thirty-two out of twenty-one thousand genes have been implicated in weight management. The difference between someone at the top of the genetic lottery and someone at the bottom is roughly seven and a half kilograms. That is not nothing, but it does not explain a country where obesity rates have gone from 1.5% in 1966 (the year I was born, the year we won the World Cup) to 28% today. In just my lifetime so far, we have put on an average of over 2 stone in weight, more weight gain than in the rest of history combined! Our genes have not changed in sixty years. Our food has.

• • •

The Liver: The Canary in the Coal Mine

Before diabetes shows up on your HbA1c, before your blood sugar is visibly out of control, there is an early warning system that almost nobody is paying attention to. Your liver.

Your liver is one of the first organs to be affected by chronically elevated insulin. When insulin is high, the liver starts storing excess glucose as fat. This is the beginning of non-alcoholic fatty liver disease, or NAFLD, and it is now one of the most common conditions in the developed world. One in four children in the UK now have fatty liver disease. Children. Sixty years ago, the condition was virtually unknown in this age group.

When your doctor checks your liver, they typically measure two enzymes called *AST* and *ALT*. If these are elevated, it means your liver cells are under stress. The problem is that the reference ranges used to define "normal" are far too lenient. In the UK, a result of up to 30 for women and up to 50 for men is considered fine. But in Isabella's KetoSAge study, the genuinely healthy participants had levels below 14. That means your doctor could look at a result of 25, tell you your liver is perfectly healthy, and miss early fatty liver disease entirely.

And in the KetoSAge study, liver markers rose significantly in just three weeks of following the UK government's dietary guidelines. Three weeks. When the participants returned to their ketogenic diet, the markers returned to baseline. The liver damage was real, measurable, and rapid. But it was also reversible.

The liver is the canary in the coal mine. It is trying to tell you something long before diabetes officially arrives. But the reference ranges are set so wide that the warning goes unheard.

The Catch-22

I covered this briefly in the heart disease chapter, but it deserves more attention here because it is so directly relevant to diabetes.

The UK government's Eatwell Guide recommends approximately 50% of your food is carbohydrates. Your liver already produces around one hundred and seventy grams of glucose per day on its own, without you eating a single thing. It does this through a process called *gluconeogenesis*. That endogenous production is enough to maintain the one teaspoon of blood sugar that your body needs.

So, the government guidelines are effectively asking you to more than double the glucose circulating in your bloodstream. On top of what your liver is already making. Every single day.

The result? Constant elevated insulin. Which suppresses your natural GLP-1 production, the very hormone that controls your appetite and makes you feel satisfied after a meal. So, you feel hungry. You eat more. More insulin is produced. More GLP-1 is suppressed. You get hungrier still.

And then, when you inevitably develop insulin resistance and start gaining weight, the same government that recommended the guidelines now funds your doctor to prescribe a GLP-1 injection. A synthetic replacement for the hormone that the government's own dietary advice suppressed in the first place.

I am not being conspiratorial. I am simply describing what the evidence shows. The guidelines drive the disease. The disease drives the prescription. And both the food industry and the pharmaceutical industry profit from the cycle. The person who loses is you.

• • •

Reversal, Not Management

Here is the part of this chapter that matters most. Type 2 diabetes and fatty liver disease are reversible. Not in every case. Not overnight. And not without effort. But the evidence is overwhelming that by addressing insulin resistance directly, through dietary changes that lower insulin, most people with type 2 diabetes or fatty liver disease can significantly improve their condition. Most can achieve blood sugar levels so normal that their medication becomes unnecessary.

But most people never try. The moment the diagnosis lands, the prescription follows, and the conversation ends there. "The medication is working, so why would I change anything?" It is one of the most common things people say, and one of the most dangerous. Because the medication is managing your blood sugar. It is not reversing the underlying insulin resistance that caused the problem. That is still there, silently doing damage. And the damage is not limited to diabetes. As you have read throughout this book, unmanaged insulin resistance increases your risk of cancer, Alzheimer's, and heart disease. But type 2 diabetes itself, when it is not properly controlled, carries its own brutal consequences. It can take your eyesight. It can cost you your feet. And research shows that for every year it is not well managed, you lose on average 100 days of life. Not quality of life. Life.

The approach is not complicated. Reduce the carbohydrates that are constantly spiking your insulin. Replace them with healthy fats and quality protein that do not trigger the same insulin response. Give your pancreas a rest. Let your cells recover their sensitivity. Allow your liver to clear the accumulated fat.

This is not a fad diet. It is a return to the way human beings ate for millions of years before processed food, before industrial agriculture, before the dietary guidelines that have coincided with the worst epidemic of metabolic disease in human history.

In the KetoSAge study, every marker that worsened on the government guidelines reversed when the participants returned to a low-carbohydrate diet. Insulin came down. IGF-1 dropped. GLP-1 recovered. Liver markers normalised. And this happened in healthy women who had only spent three weeks eating the recommended diet. The damage was quick. The recovery was quicker.

Imagine what is possible for someone who has spent twenty years eating that way, if they are willing to make the change.

• • •

My Dad

He was diagnosed with type 2 diabetes after decades of eating the way his generation was told to eat. Plenty of bread, potatoes, cereal, and fruit juice. Low fat where possible. Margarine instead of butter. All the things the guidelines recommended.

He was given medication. He was told to manage his condition. Nobody ever told him it was reversible. Nobody ever suggested that the food itself might be the problem, or that changing it might be the solution.

I cannot change what happened to my dad. But I wrote this chapter for everyone who is in the position he was in. Everyone who has been told that diabetes is a life sentence. Everyone who has been given bigger buckets instead of being shown where the pipe is burst.

It is not your fault. The system that created this crisis is the same system that profits from it. But now you know. And knowing is the first step towards taking back control.

CHAPTER EIGHT

The Hidden Damage

• • •

In the previous chapters we looked at the big four. Cancer. Alzheimer's. Heart disease. Diabetes. These are the diseases that fill the headlines and dominate the conversations in hospital waiting rooms. They are the ones that frighten people the most. And rightly so.

But insulin resistance does not stop there. Not even close.

Take another look at my *Tree of Afflictions* and you will see that insulin resistance sits at the trunk and the diseases branch outwards. The big four are the thickest branches. But there are dozens of smaller branches, and each one represents a condition that is quietly damaging millions of lives. Some of them you will have heard of. Some of them you might be living with right now without ever connecting them to your diet.

This chapter is about those smaller branches. The conditions that rarely make the front page but are just as rooted in the same soil. The hidden damage that insulin resistance does to your body while everyone is looking the other way.

• • •

Gout: Not What You Think

My dad has been a long-time warrior against gout. It has been shadowing him for years, an unwelcome companion that flares up without warning and leaves him barely able to walk.

Most people think of gout as an old-fashioned disease. Something that affected Henry VIII from too much port and red meat. The reality is very different. Gout has surged by 29% between 1997 and 2012 in the UK alone. That is not a disease of kings. That is an epidemic.

The mechanism is one we have seen before. Under normal circumstances, uric acid is efficiently cleared by the kidneys and excreted in your urine. But insulin resistance disrupts that process. The kidneys start retaining uric acid instead of expelling it. Levels build in the bloodstream and eventually the uric acid crystallises in your joints, most commonly in the big toe, but also in the ankles, fingers and wrists. Those crystals trigger a vicious inflammatory response, and the result is the redness, swelling and excruciating pain that anyone who has experienced gout will know all too well.

But here is the twist. While we often point the finger at glucose for insulin problems, with gout the spotlight turns to a different culprit: fructose. The same fructose found in the orange juice and apple juice that we hand our children every morning. The same fructose that the food industry pours into soft drinks and processed foods. The rise in gout tracks almost perfectly alongside the rise in fructose consumption, obesity and insulin resistance. They are all expressions of the same underlying problem.

My dad's doctor treated his gout as a standalone condition. Gave him medication to manage the uric acid. Never once mentioned insulin. Never once connected it to his blood pressure, his blood sugar, or anything else on the tree. Every branch was treated as a separate tree. That is the fundamental failure.

• • •

Erectile Dysfunction and the Conversation Nobody Wants to Have

This is one of those topics that people avoid, but it is too important to skip. Erectile dysfunction affects a huge number of men, and the numbers are rising in younger age groups every decade. The standard response is a prescription for Viagra or similar medication, and the conversation ends there.

But erectile dysfunction is, in many cases, an early warning sign that something much deeper is going wrong. It is a vascular condition. The blood vessels that supply the penis are some of the smallest in the body, and when insulin resistance begins to damage the endothelium, the lining of those blood vessels, the smallest vessels fail first. In that sense, erectile dysfunction can be one of the earliest detectable signs of cardiovascular damage. It is your body sending a signal that all is not well.

We know from the science discussed in earlier chapters that excess insulin damages endothelial cells, thickens arterial walls, and increases blood viscosity. We know it triggers aromatase, which converts testosterone into oestrogen, disrupting the hormonal balance that men depend on. And we know that high insulin suppresses the production of nitric oxide, which is essential for healthy blood flow.

My dad, bless him, had gout, then came the high blood pressure, then came the discreet nod to Viagra. Each one treated as a separate problem. Each one managed with a separate prescription. Nobody joined the dots.

If you are a man experiencing erectile dysfunction, please do not just accept a prescription and move on. Ask your doctor to test your fasting insulin. Because the blood vessel damage that is affecting you there is the same damage that may, in time, affect your heart and your brain. Once again, it's the insulin problem.

PCOS, Fertility, and the Crisis Nobody Is Talking About

Polycystic ovary syndrome, or PCOS, is the number one cause of infertility in women. And according to both Professor Ben Bikman and Dr Isabella Cooper, the number one cause of PCOS is hyperinsulinaemia. Elevated insulin.

"Elevated insulin and hyperinsulinaemia are the number one cause for PCOS. PCOS is the number one cause for females not having children or infertility." Ben Bikman

PCOS is a hormonal condition that disrupts ovulation and can cause a cascade of symptoms including irregular periods, weight gain, acne, and excess hair growth. It is typically managed with hormonal contraceptives or metformin, but the root cause is rarely addressed. And the root cause, in the overwhelming majority of cases, is too much insulin circulating in the blood, throwing the entire hormonal system off balance.

As Ben Bikman has explained to me, here is the cruel twist: while most of your body's cells eventually stop listening to insulin and become resistant, the ovaries do not. The theca cells in your ovaries remain sensitive to insulin even when other parts of your body have shut the door. So, when insulin levels are chronically elevated, those cells keep responding. They get bombarded with signals to produce androgens, the male hormones like testosterone, and they oblige. The result is an overproduction of androgens that disrupts ovulation, drives the symptoms of PCOS, and in about 80% of cases makes conception extraordinarily difficult. The ovaries are, in effect, one of the last tissues still taking insulin's calls, and they are paying the price for it.

But the fertility crisis runs deeper than PCOS alone. Isabella painted a picture during our conversation that genuinely alarmed me. She explained that when you are hyperinsulinaemic, conditions like autism spectrum disorder and ADHD become more pronounced. These conditions create difficulty in social interaction. And we need young people socially interacting in order to form relationships and eventually have families:

"High carbs, high insulin. That is actually the downfall of mankind in the end, if we are not producing enough offspring."

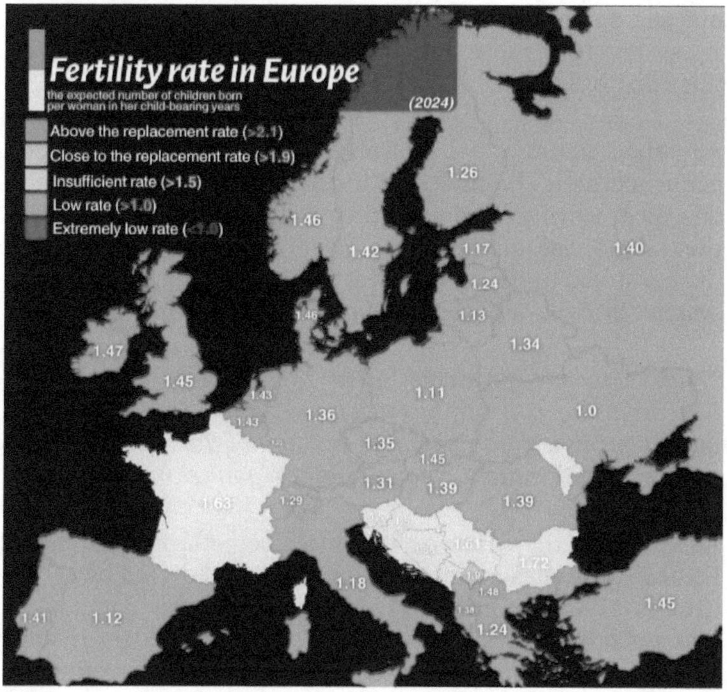

Fertility rates in Europe

We are not exaggerating here. Take a look at the chart above. It shows the number of children being born across Europe. Not a single country is now achieving the 2.1 children per woman needed to sustain its population. High-carbohydrate diets lead to insulin resistance. Insulin resistance leads to erectile dysfunction and PCOS. And now, not one European nation is producing enough children to maintain its natural population. That is not a coincidence. That is cause and effect.

Then Isabella raised something else that most people never consider. Epigenetic imprinting. When a mother has high insulin during pregnancy, the child is born with a predisposition to produce more insulin. That child grows up in the same food environment, eats the same high-carbohydrate diet, and the cycle deepens with each generation. We are not just damaging ourselves. We are programming the next generation to be more susceptible before they have even taken their first breath.

And then there is the environmental layer. Isabella spoke about synthetic clothing, plastics, skincare products and seed oils, all of which contain compounds that mimic oestrogen in the body. These add to the methylation burden, contribute to the hormonal traffic jam, and further disrupt the reproductive system. Isabella echoed what I have already written:

"With skincare products, plus toothpastes, makeup, in fact anything you apply to your skin, when you read the ingredient list, if you wouldn't eat any of the ingredients or can't pronounce them, do not put it on your skin."

Add it all together, and you start to see something frightening. Falling birth rates are not just a social trend driven by career choices and economics. There is a biological component that nobody in government wants to acknowledge. Insulin resistance is directly undermining our ability to reproduce as a species. And we are making it worse with every generation.

• • •

Shortened Telomeres and the Ageing Question

There is one more item on the tree that deserves attention, because it touches all of us: shortened telomeres.

Telomeres are the protective caps on the ends of your chromosomes, a bit like the plastic tips on the ends of shoelaces. Every time a cell divides, the telomeres shorten slightly. When they get too short, the cell can no longer divide properly and it either dies or becomes dysfunctional. The length of your telomeres is one of the most reliable biological markers of ageing. Longer telomeres are associated with better health and longer life. Shorter telomeres are associated with accelerated ageing and disease.

And what shortens telomeres prematurely? Chronic inflammation. Oxidative stress. Excess insulin. The very conditions that insulin resistance creates. The *m*TOR pathway, which we discussed in the cancer chapter, plays a role here too. When *m*TOR is permanently switched on by chronically elevated insulin, cells are constantly being pushed to grow and divide rather than entering repair mode. That accelerated division burns through telomere length faster than it should.

In other words, insulin resistance does not just make you ill. It makes you age faster. The diseases on the tree are not just separate medical problems. They are expressions of a body that is wearing out ahead of schedule because the repair systems have been overwhelmed and the growth signals never switch off.

Autophagy, the cellular housekeeping process we discussed earlier, is one of the body's primary mechanisms for slowing this down. When insulin is low and *m*TOR is quiet, autophagy kicks in and clears out damaged cells and cellular debris. But when insulin is permanently elevated, autophagy is suppressed. The rubbish accumulates. The telomeres shorten.

And you age, not at the pace nature intended, but at the pace that your diet dictates.

• • •

Osteoporosis: It Is Not a Calcium Problem

Most people think of osteoporosis as a calcium deficiency. Drink more milk. Take a supplement. That is the extent of the advice. But osteoporosis is not a calcium problem. It is a metabolic problem. And once you understand the role insulin plays, the standard advice starts to look dangerously incomplete.

In the UK, one in two women and one in five men over 50 will suffer an osteoporotic fracture in their lifetime. Hip fractures alone account for thousands of deaths each year, and for those who survive, the loss of independence can be devastating.

Here is what your doctor is unlikely to tell you. Chronically elevated insulin and the cortisol that accompanies a stressed, inflamed body both cause calcium to leach from your bones. You can take all the calcium supplements you like, but if your insulin is chronically high, your body is pulling calcium out faster than you can put it back in. It is like filling a bath with the plug out.

There is another layer to this. Insulin drives the *m*TOR pathway, which as we have already discussed pushes cells into constant growth mode at the expense of repair. Bone is living tissue. It is constantly being broken down by cells called osteoclasts and rebuilt by cells called osteoblasts. In a healthy body, this process is balanced. But when insulin is chronically elevated and inflammation is running unchecked, the breakdown accelerates and the rebuilding falls behind. Your bones are being dismantled faster than they are being repaired.

Post-menopausal women are hit hardest, and it is no coincidence that this is also the point at which insulin resistance tends to accelerate. As oestrogen drops, the protective metabolic effects it provided start to disappear. Insulin resistance that may have been quietly building for decades suddenly has free rein. The bones, already under metabolic stress, begin to deteriorate rapidly.

Weight-bearing exercise is genuinely protective, because it stimulates the osteoblasts to build new bone. But the other half of the equation, the one that rarely gets mentioned, is addressing the insulin. Reducing carbohydrates, lowering chronic inflammation, and giving your body the metabolic environment it needs to rebuild rather than just break down. That is not a conversation most osteoporosis clinics are having. But it should be.

• • •

Parkinson's Disease: The Dopamine Connection

Parkinson's disease is typically described as a condition where the brain stops producing enough dopamine, the neurotransmitter that controls movement, mood, and motivation. The tremors, the rigidity, the shuffling gait, these are all consequences of dopamine depletion. What is rarely discussed is why the dopamine disappears in the first place.

The numbers tell a story. Up to 80% of people with Parkinson's disease also display insulin resistance or type 2 diabetes. That is not a footnote. That is the majority of patients sharing the same underlying metabolic dysfunction that drives every other condition in this book.

Research has shown that elevated insulin casts a direct shadow over dopamine production. A 2015 study published by Andre

Kleinridders and colleagues found that insulin resistance in the brain alters dopamine turnover and causes behavioural disorders. When insulin is high, the dopamine system suffers. When insulin is reduced, dopamine receptors increase. The relationship is not subtle.

The brain cells that produce dopamine, located in an area called the substantia nigra, are packed with mitochondria. They have to be, because producing dopamine is an energy-intensive process. And as we have discussed throughout this book, chronically elevated insulin damages mitochondria. It drives oxidative stress. It suppresses autophagy, the repair process that would normally clear out damaged cellular components before they cause problems. When the mitochondria in these dopamine-producing cells fail, the cells fail with them.

In a small but striking study, five out of seven Parkinson's patients placed on a ketogenic diet saw measurable improvements within a single month. Better cognitive function. Less pain. Less fatigue. Improved sleep. These were patients for whom conventional medication had offered limited relief. Nobody is suggesting a ketogenic diet is a cure for Parkinson's. But the fact that changing fuel, from glucose to ketones, could improve symptoms in four weeks should be making every neurologist in the country sit up and pay attention.

It is the same pattern we see everywhere. The brain needs energy. Insulin resistance compromises that energy supply. The most vulnerable cells, the ones working hardest, fail first. In Alzheimer's it is the memory centres. In Parkinson's it is the dopamine factories. Different symptoms, same root cause.

And yet, when a patient walks into a neurology clinic with early Parkinson's, nobody asks what they eat. Nobody measures their insulin. Nobody connects the tremor in their hand to the toast and orange juice they had for breakfast. The branches are treated. The trunk is ignored.

Peripheral Neuropathy: When Your Nerves Stop Listening

One in ten people in the UK are affected by some degree of peripheral neuropathy. That is the numbness, tingling, and burning pain that typically starts in the feet and hands and can gradually spread. It can also disrupt digestion, bladder function, and blood pressure regulation. For many people, it is a constant, grinding discomfort that erodes their quality of life.

Most doctors associate peripheral neuropathy with advanced diabetes. It is considered a complication of the disease, something that happens after years of poorly controlled blood sugar. And that is true, as far as it goes. But it does not go nearly far enough.

Nerve cells have insulin receptors. They are responsive to insulin, and they depend on it for normal function. As those nerve cells become insulin resistant, their ability to maintain themselves deteriorates. The myelin sheath, the protective coating around the nerve fibre that allows signals to travel quickly and cleanly, begins to break down. Signals slow. Signals distort. Eventually, signals stop altogether.

The damage does not wait for a diabetes diagnosis. It begins with insulin resistance, years or even decades before blood sugar rises high enough to trigger an HbA1c flag. A person can have perfectly normal blood sugar, because their pancreas is still compensating, while their nerves are already quietly deteriorating. By the time the tingling starts, the damage has been accumulating for a long time.

There is a cruel irony here. The smallest nerve fibres are the ones affected first. These are the nerves responsible for sensing temperature, pain, and light touch. They are also the nerves that monitor the health of your blood vessels. When they fail, you lose the early warning system that would otherwise alert you to vascular damage. The very damage that insulin resistance is causing elsewhere in your body.

This is why peripheral neuropathy is not just a nuisance. It is a signal. If you are experiencing numbness or tingling in your feet, it is not just your nerves telling you something is wrong. It is your metabolism. And the question your doctor should be asking is not how to manage the symptoms, but what is driving the insulin resistance that is causing them.

• • •

Osteoarthritis: Not Just Wear and Tear

If you mention osteoarthritis to most people, they will tell you it is caused by getting old, being overweight, or overdoing it at the gym. Wear and tear. That is the phrase you hear in every GP surgery in the country. And it is wrong.

Ten million people in the UK live with osteoarthritis. Six million are women. Four million are men. It is one of the leading causes of disability. And the standard treatment is painkillers, anti-inflammatories, and eventually joint replacement surgery. Nobody looks upstream.

Before we go further, it is worth understanding that there are two main types of arthritis and they are very different conditions. Rheumatoid arthritis is an autoimmune disease where your immune system attacks the lining of your joints. It can strike at any age and tends to affect both sides of the body symmetrically. Osteoarthritis is the breakdown of cartilage, the smooth, protective surface that cushions your joints. It is far more common, affecting ten times as many people, and it is the one we are focusing on here. What they have in common, and what most doctors overlook, is that both are strongly linked to insulin resistance and chronic inflammation.

But both osteoarthritis and insulin resistance share common ground at the cellular level. The cartilage in your joints is maintained by cells called chondrocytes. These cells depend on a stable metabolic environment to do their job, building, repairing, and maintaining the smooth, shock-absorbing surface that allows your joints to move freely. When that metabolic environment is disrupted by chronically elevated insulin, everything changes.

Insulin resistance drives low-grade systemic inflammation. That inflammation does not just affect your arteries or your liver. It attacks your cartilage. It alters glucose and lipid metabolism in the chondrocytes, disrupting the delicate balance between cartilage repair and cartilage breakdown. And it increases oxidative stress, the same reactive oxygen species we discussed earlier, which directly damages joint tissue.

This is why osteoarthritis correlates so strongly with insulin resistance, even in joints that bear no weight at all. If it were simply wear and tear, you would expect it only in knees and hips. But osteoarthritis also appears in hands, wrists, and fingers, joints that carry no body weight whatsoever. That makes no sense if the cause is mechanical. It makes perfect sense if the cause is metabolic.

Visceral fat, the deep belly fat that is a hallmark of insulin resistance, is particularly problematic. It does not just sit there. It is metabolically active, pumping out inflammatory cytokines that circulate through your entire body, including your joints. Every kilogram of visceral fat is a factory producing the very chemicals that degrade your cartilage.

There is another mechanism at work here that very few people know about, and it connects directly to the liver. If you are carrying a lot of visceral fat, you will almost certainly have a fatty liver to some degree. A fatty liver triggers the overproduction of an enzyme called matrix metalloproteinases, or MMPs. In a healthy body, MMPs break down proteins that provide structural support for your cells and aid wound healing. But a fatty liver generates an overexpression of these enzymes, and the body has to send the excess somewhere. They end up gathering in your joints, particularly in the lower body: hips and knees. MMPs are one of the only enzymes in the body that can actually attack your joints' connective tissue, the extracellular matrix that your joints are made of. They literally degrade the structure from the inside.

I speak from experience. I took up tennis at 40, and for the best part of a decade I was carrying too much weight and my knees were a constant problem. Pain, swelling, the sort of nagging discomfort that makes you question whether you should be playing at all. Once I lost the weight and got my metabolic health in order, the knee problems virtually disappeared. I rarely have any issues now. My knees did not change. My diet did.

So, if you are experiencing ongoing knee or hip pain and you are overweight, you may not have an injury or arthritis at all. You may have a metabolic problem. The pain is not coming from wear and tear. It is coming from your liver. Fix the diet, reduce the fatty liver, reduce the MMP overproduction, and the joint degradation begins to slow. I would not be surprised if a significant number of people currently on the waiting list for a hip or knee replacement could avoid the operating table entirely by addressing their insulin resistance and reversing their fatty liver disease first. But nobody is testing for it. They are just handing out painkillers and booking surgery.

• • •

Acid Reflux and Tinnitus

I want to touch briefly on a handful of conditions that most people would never connect to their diet, let alone to insulin resistance.

Take acid reflux. One in four people in the UK suffer from it. The standard advice is to avoid fatty food, cut back on coffee, and take an antacid. But Dr Norman Robillard's work has shown that the real mechanism is far more interesting. Cycles of carbohydrate malabsorption lead to bacterial overgrowth in the small intestine, which produces gas, which propels acid upwards. It is not too much acid. It is gas pressure from the wrong bacteria being fed the wrong food. Fix the diet, restore the microbiome, and for many people the reflux disappears.

Then there is tinnitus, that persistent ringing or buzzing in the ears that drives people to distraction. Most people assume it is an ear problem, and it is, but the underlying driver is chronic inflammation within the ear. A study from the Federal University of Rio Grande in Brazil found that 84 to 92% of people suffering from tinnitus were hyperinsulinaemic. The inner ear runs directly on glucose supplied by the blood. When glucose metabolism is disrupted, the delicate workings of the inner ear are thrown off balance. Fix the insulin, reduce the inflammation, and the ringing often fades.

• • •

Migraines: Your Brain Running on Empty

Migraines affect roughly 12% of the world's population. They are the leading cause of disability in people under 50 and in 2016 alone were responsible for an estimated 45 million years of life lived in pain. Most people treat them with painkillers and wait for them to pass. Very few ask why they happen.

The emerging science suggests that migraines are, at least in part, a metabolic event. Your brain is an energy-hungry organ. When insulin resistance disrupts glucose delivery to the brain, the cells do not simply go quiet. They protest. Professor Ben Bikman describes it as a "running on empty" scenario, where the brain, starved of its primary fuel, triggers a cascade of inflammation and swelling as it tries to reset itself. It is not a headache. It is an energy crisis.

This is why a growing body of research points to a ketogenic diet as one of the most effective interventions. In one clinical trial, 50 migraine patients were placed on a ketogenic diet for three months. Both the severity and the frequency of their migraines dropped dramatically. By switching the brain's fuel from glucose to ketones, the energy supply becomes more stable, the inflammation quiets down, and the migraines lose their trigger.

I am not suggesting everyone with migraines needs to go keto. Stress, poor sleep, caffeine, alcohol, and hormonal changes are all legitimate triggers and should be addressed first. But if you have tried everything else and the migraines persist, the question worth asking is this: is your brain getting the fuel it needs? Because if insulin resistance is blocking that fuel, no painkiller in the world will fix the cause.

• • •

Menopause and Insulin Resistance

Menopause typically occurs when a woman has not had a period for twelve consecutive months, usually between the ages of 40 and 55. It is a natural transition, driven by a decline in oestrogen production. But what most women are not told is that this hormonal shift does not just affect their reproductive system. It affects their metabolic system too.

Oestrogen plays a protective role in insulin sensitivity. While it is present, it helps your cells respond to insulin efficiently. When oestrogen drops during menopause, that protection disappears. Professor Ben Bikman has highlighted compelling evidence that oestrogen, in both men and women, helps maintain insulin sensitivity. People whose bodies cannot produce oestrogen due to a deficiency in the enzyme aromatase develop insulin resistance as a direct consequence.

This is why so many women experience weight gain, fatigue, and rising blood sugar around menopause, even when their diet has not changed. The food is the same. The hormonal environment is not. Insulin resistance that may have been quietly building for years suddenly accelerates once oestrogen is no longer holding it in check.

For some women, hormone replacement therapy provides meaningful relief. For others, dietary change is the more effective lever. What matters is understanding that the weight gain and metabolic disruption of menopause are not inevitable consequences of ageing. They are consequences of insulin resistance meeting a hormonal cliff edge. Address the insulin, and many of the symptoms become manageable.

• • •

Menstrual Pain: The Inflammation Connection

Painful periods are the leading cause of school absence among teenage girls, and up to 90% of menstruating women experience them to some degree. The medical term is dysmenorrhoea, and the standard response is ibuprofen and a hot water bottle.

But the severity of menstrual cramps is driven in large part by prostaglandins, hormone-like chemicals that ramp up inflammation and trigger uterine contractions. The more inflamed your body already is, the more prostaglandins you produce, and the worse the pain.

This is where diet comes in. A diet high in sugar, seed oils, and ultra-processed food drives chronic low-grade inflammation throughout the body. That inflammation does not pause during menstruation. It amplifies it. Reducing sugar spikes by eating fibre first, cutting back on seed oils, and increasing omega-3 intake can all lower the baseline level of inflammation in your body and, with it, the severity of menstrual pain.

This is not a replacement for medical advice. Conditions like endometriosis and fibroids can intensify menstrual pain and need proper investigation. But for the millions of women whose pain has no identified underlying cause, the question is worth asking: is your diet driving the inflammation that is making your periods worse?

• • •

Leaky Gut: When the Barrier Breaks Down

Your gut lining is designed to be selectively permeable. It lets water and nutrients through while keeping bacteria, toxins, and undigested food particles out. When that lining is damaged, the barrier becomes too permeable, a condition commonly called leaky gut, and the consequences ripple across your entire body.

The primary dietary drivers are a lack of fibre and an excess of fructose. Fructose, the sugar found in fruit juice, soft drinks, and most processed foods, has been shown to loosen the tight junctions between the cells of the intestinal wall. Once those junctions open, bacterial fragments and other unwanted molecules slip into the bloodstream and trigger an immune response. That immune response shows up as chronic low-grade inflammation, the same inflammation that drives insulin resistance and feeds every condition on the tree.

Fibre does the opposite. It feeds the beneficial bacteria in your gut, which in turn produce short-chain fatty acids. Those fatty acids strengthen the mucin layer that coats your intestinal wall and reinforce the tight junctions that hold the barrier together. In simple terms: fibre builds the wall up. Fructose and processed food knock it down.

This is also why leaky gut and insulin resistance so often travel together. The inflammation caused by a compromised gut barrier makes insulin resistance worse. The insulin resistance drives further dietary choices that damage the gut. It is a self-reinforcing cycle, and breaking it starts with the same intervention as nearly everything else in this book: fix what you eat.

• • •

Acne: The Skin's Insulin Signal

95% of people between 11 and 30 experience acne. It is so common that most people treat it as a normal part of growing up rather than a symptom of something deeper. But acne is, in many cases, a visible marker of what is happening to your insulin.

When blood sugar spikes, the body releases insulin. That insulin triggers the production of insulin-like growth factor 1 (IGF-1), which pushes the sebaceous glands in your skin into overdrive. They produce excess sebum, the oily substance that clogs pores and creates the perfect environment for acne. At the same time, elevated insulin drives androgen production, the same hormonal disruption we discussed in the PCOS section, and androgens further stimulate oil production and inflammation in the skin.

In one study, young men with and without acne were given glucose-laden drinks. The insulin response in acne sufferers was dramatically higher, quadrupling in overweight participants and doubling in leaner ones. The skin was not causing the problem. The insulin was.

My friend Christian Dailly, a personal trainer who works with young athletes, has observed the same thing from the practical side. When his clients switch to a low-carbohydrate diet, their skin clears up. Not after months of treatment. Within weeks. Nobody prescribed a cream. They just changed what they ate.

• • •

Eczema: Another Branch, Same Root

Eczema is subtler than acne but no less connected to what is happening inside your body. Those itchy, inflamed patches are driven by immune dysfunction and chronic inflammation, both of which are amplified by insulin resistance and a damaged gut.

Ultra-processed foods and gluten are among the most commonly reported dietary triggers, though eczema is highly individual and what provokes it in one person may be harmless to another. Stress, skincare products, synthetic clothing and environmental factors all play their part.

But the metabolic thread is consistent. A diet that drives inflammation, disrupts the gut microbiome, and keeps insulin elevated creates the conditions in which eczema thrives. Address those underlying drivers, reduce the sugar, increase the fibre, repair the gut, and for many people the skin begins to calm.

Acne and eczema are not just cosmetic complaints. They are your skin broadcasting what your metabolism is doing beneath the surface. Listen to it.

Every condition in this chapter sits on a branch of the *Tree of Afflictions*. Every one of them has a documented connection to insulin resistance and chronic inflammation. And every one of them is routinely treated as an isolated condition with its own specialist, its own prescription, and its own waiting list.

Nobody steps back and sees the tree.

CHAPTER NINE

The Immune System Nobody Talks About

• • •

If I asked you where your immune system lives, most people would shrug and say something about white blood cells floating around in the blood. Maybe they would mention the lymph nodes. A few might point to the thymus gland if they paid attention in biology. Almost nobody would point to their gut.

And yet, approximately 80% of your entire immune system resides in your gut. 80%. That is not a typo. The vast majority of your body's defence force is stationed in and around your digestive tract, intertwined with a community of trillions of microorganisms that collectively make up your microbiome. These microscopic residents, your bacteria, viruses, fungi and other microbial partners, are not passengers. They are active participants in your health. They train your immune cells. They regulate inflammation. They produce compounds that protect you from disease. And when they are healthy and diverse, you are healthier and more resilient than you could ever be without them.

This chapter is about a symbiotic relationship. Because insulin resistance does not just damage your organs and hormones. It damages the ecosystem inside you that keeps everything else in check. And when that ecosystem falls apart, so does your ability to fight back.

• • •

A City Inside You

To understand how profoundly your microbiome affects your health, you need to appreciate its scale. Only about 10% of the cells in your body are actually human. The other 90% belong to your microbial community. In the human gut alone, there are over 140,000 different variants of viruses and close to 2,000 species of bacteria. There are over 260 species of fungi.

I like to call these inhabitants our "Microbial Partners", because the word bacteria tends to create a negative image, and that is not fair. Most of them are on our side. Of the millions of different microscopic life forms on this planet, only around 400 have any conflict with humans, and just 150 pose a risk of causing widespread disease. The overwhelming majority are allies.

Think of your gut as a bustling coral reef. When conditions are right, when the water is clean and the nutrients are balanced, the reef thrives with extraordinary diversity. Thousands of species coexist, each playing their part. But when conditions deteriorate, when the temperature shifts or pollution creeps in, the most vulnerable species vanish first. Hardy, opportunistic organisms take over. The reef loses its colour, its complexity, its resilience. What is left looks alive, but it is a shadow of what it was.

That is precisely what happens inside your gut when your diet is wrong. When you strip the fibre out, flood the system with sugar and ultra-processed food, and bombard it with antibiotics and antibacterial products, the diverse ecosystem starts to collapse. The beneficial species retreat. The less helpful ones, particularly a group of bacteria called Firmicutes, rush in to fill the gap. And with that shift comes a cascade of consequences that reach far beyond your digestive system.

• • •

Firmicutes, Bacteroidetes, and the Weight Connection

Before we go further, I want to tell you about two families of bacteria that have an extraordinary influence on your body weight.

In 2004, Professor Fredrik Backhed at the University of Gothenburg in Sweden conducted a remarkable experiment. He took skinny mice that had been born by caesarean section and raised in a completely sterile environment, with no gut bacteria at all. He then took bacteria from the gut of obese mice and introduced it to these sterile animals. Within weeks, without changing their diet at all, the previously lean mice became obese, packing on an average of 60% more weight. Even when the professor reduced their food intake, the mice continued to gain weight.

Later, a human study took bacteria from two twin sisters, one lean and one obese, and introduced each set of bacteria into separate groups of mice. The mice that received bacteria from the obese twin became obese. The mice that received bacteria from the lean twin stayed lean. Same food. Different microbiome. Different outcome.

The difference comes down to these two bacterial families. Firmicutes are experts at extracting every possible calorie from your food. The more Firmicutes you have, the more energy your body absorbs, and the more weight you carry. Bacteroidetes do the opposite. They extract the essential nutrients and vitamins and then allow excess calories to pass through, carried out in your stool on the back of dietary fibre.

Now here is the critical point. What feeds and promotes Bacteroidetes? Fibre. What starves Bacteroidetes and allows Firmicutes to dominate? A diet stripped of fibre, loaded with sugar and refined carbohydrates. In other words, the modern Western diet. If you have struggled with your weight and felt that it could not simply be explained by how much you eat, you may be right. The composition of your microbiome, shaped by what you eat, may be doing as much to determine your body weight as the calories on your plate.

• • •

Short-Chain Fatty Acids: Your Gut's Secret Weapon

When your good bacteria eat fibre, they do not just sit quietly and digest it. They transform it into something remarkable: short-chain fatty acids, or SCFAs. These are small but extraordinarily powerful molecules, and they are the real currency of gut health.

There are three main SCFAs that matter: butyrate, acetate and propionate. Between them, they perform a list of functions that would make any pharmaceutical company weep with envy.

Butyrate is the star of the show. Around 70% of the energy used by your colon cells comes directly from butyrate. Without it, those cells struggle to maintain themselves. But butyrate does far more than feed the colon. It strengthens the tight junctions that hold your gut lining together, preventing the leaky gut syndrome we have already discussed. It suppresses inflammation within the gut. It directly combats harmful bacteria like salmonella and E. coli. And it sends signals to your immune system that help it distinguish between genuine threats and harmless substances.

Acetate and propionate play supporting roles that are just as important. Acetate helps regulate appetite. Propionate influences cholesterol metabolism and has anti-inflammatory properties. Together, the three create a self-sustaining cycle: the more fibre you eat, the more good bacteria thrive. The more good bacteria thrive, the more SCFAs they produce. The more SCFAs they produce, the healthier your gut lining, the calmer your inflammation, and the stronger your immune response.

Now think about what happens when that cycle breaks. When there is no fibre to feed the good bacteria, SCFA production drops. The gut lining weakens. Inflammation rises. The immune system loses its training ground. And the whole defence network begins to crumble from the inside.

• • •

When the Immune System Turns on Itself

A healthy, well-trained immune system is a precision instrument. It identifies genuine threats, mobilises the right cells to the right location, neutralises the danger, and stands down. It knows the difference between a harmful invader and a piece of harmless pollen or a molecule of food protein.

A poorly trained immune system is a blunt weapon. It overreacts. It misidentifies. It attacks things it should ignore and, in the worst cases, it turns on your own body.

That is what autoimmune disease is. Your immune system, confused and dysregulated, begins attacking your own tissues as if they were foreign invaders. Type 1 diabetes, where the immune system destroys the insulin-producing cells in the pancreas. Multiple sclerosis, where it attacks the protective coating around nerve fibres. Crohn's disease, where it wages war on the digestive tract itself. Rheumatoid arthritis, where it targets the joints. Lupus, coeliac disease, eczema, psoriasis. The list is long and growing.

Since the 1950s, rates of type 1 diabetes, multiple sclerosis and Crohn's disease have risen by 300% or more. 300%. That is not a gradual drift. That is an explosion. And it maps almost exactly onto the period in which our diets shifted towards ultra-processed food, our antibiotic use skyrocketed, and our obsession with antibacterial products intensified.

• • •

Allergies: Friendly Fire

Allergies are the immune system's version of friendly fire. Instead of attacking a genuine pathogen, the immune system overreacts to something harmless: pollen, dust, pet hair, certain foods. The result is the runny nose, the itchy eyes, the wheezing, the skin reactions, and in severe cases, life-threatening anaphylaxis.

Allergies have now become the most common chronic disease in Europe. It is predicted that by 2027, half of the entire EU population will suffer from some form of allergic condition. Hospital admissions for severe allergic reactions increased sevenfold between 2005 and 2015. Every waiter in every restaurant now asks if you have allergies, because the answer is increasingly likely to be yes.

Asthma has increased tenfold in the Western world since the 1960s. According to the World Health Organisation, 300 million people worldwide now suffer from it, and 250,000 die from it every year.

Why? Because your microbiome is where your immune system learns the difference between friend and foe. When the microbiome is diverse and well-fed, it trains immune cells properly. When it is impoverished and out of balance, that training breaks down. The immune system becomes jumpy, reactive, unable to tell the difference between a dangerous pathogen and a grain of pollen. The result is allergies. And, in more extreme cases, autoimmune disease.

And what impoverishes the microbiome more than anything else? A diet high in ultra-processed food and refined carbohydrates, the same diet that spikes insulin, starves your gut bacteria of fibre, and strips away the very ecosystem your immune system depends on to function properly.

• • •

Insulin, Inflammation, and the Vicious Cycle

Now let me connect all of this back to the trunk of the tree. Insulin resistance and a damaged microbiome do not just coexist. They feed each other in a vicious cycle. When your microbiome is compromised, it disrupts the balance of your gut flora, leading to inflammation. That inflammation contributes to insulin resistance. And insulin resistance, in turn, creates the metabolic conditions that further damage the microbiome. Round and round it goes.

But which one comes first? This is where a blood marker called *CRP* becomes important. *CRP* stands for *C-reactive protein*. It is produced by your liver and released into the bloodstream whenever there is inflammation in your body. Doctors use it as a general alarm signal. When *CRP* is high, something somewhere is inflamed. It is one of the most widely used markers for systemic inflammation, the kind that is not in one specific place but running through your entire system.

In Isabella's KetoSAge study, something revealing happened. When the healthy participants switched to the government's recommended high-carbohydrate diet, their liver markers worsened and insulin resistance appeared. But *CRP* did not rise. As Isabella explained:

"CRP, the marker for systemic inflammation, did not rise with the liver damage in our study. This shows insulin

resistance occurs before systemic inflammation. It is not that inflammation causes insulin resistance. Actually, insulin resistance comes first, and inflammation follows."

That finding is important because it tells us the direction of travel. Insulin resistance is not caused by inflammation. Insulin resistance causes inflammation. It is the first domino. And once that domino falls, the inflammatory cascade damages everything downstream, including the microbiome that is supposed to be keeping the inflammation in check.

This is why you cannot fix your immune system with a supplement alone. You cannot pop a probiotic capsule and expect your gut to repair itself while you continue to eat the food that destroyed it in the first place. Probiotics are the residents. But they need somewhere to live. They need prebiotics, the fibre that feeds them and creates the environment in which they can thrive. Without fibre, introducing good bacteria into a damaged gut is like planting seeds in concrete. They cannot take root.

• • •

Rebuilding What Was Lost

The good news is that your microbiome is remarkably resilient. Dr David Perlmutter reminds us that the gut microbiotic community is wonderfully receptive to rehabilitation.

Step one is fibre. This will not surprise you by now, but it bears repeating because it is the single most important thing you can do for your microbiome. Fibre is a prebiotic, the foundation, the food that your good bacteria need to survive and multiply. When you eat fibre-rich foods, you are feeding Bacteroidetes and starving Firmicutes. You are promoting the production of SCFAs. You are strengthening your gut lining. You are reducing inflammation. And you are giving your immune system the training ground it needs to function properly. Garlic and onions deserve a special mention here. They are among the richest natural sources of inulin, a type of prebiotic fibre that your beneficial bacteria thrive on. They also contain compounds with natural antimicrobial and anti-inflammatory properties. If fibre is the foundation, garlic and onions are the fertiliser.

Step two is variety. Different bacteria thrive on different fibres, and different fibres come from different foods. Dr Rob Knight, the mastermind behind the American Gut Project, the world's largest microbiome research project, concluded that food diversity is the single most important factor for a thriving microbiome. Our planet has over 290,000 edible plants, each with its own unique mix of fibres. Our ancestors ate from a staggeringly varied menu. Today, most of us rotate through the same handful of meals week after week. Your gut craves variety the way a coral reef craves biodiversity.

I should say, however, that not all scientists agree on the importance of diversification. Ben Bikman, for one, has his reservations. If you are following a ketogenic or carnivore diet and thriving, the idea that you must eat 30 different plants a week can feel like a contradiction. Ben's argument is that if your metabolic health is excellent, your inflammation is low, and your gut is functioning well, then the diversity of your food may matter less than the quality of it. It is a fair point, and an honest one. My own view is that for the majority of people, especially those still eating a standard UK diet, variety is a powerful tool. But if you have already removed the foods that were causing the damage in the first place, the rules may look different.

Step three is to stop the destruction. Reduce your use of antibacterial products outside of genuine medical necessity. Think twice about unnecessary antibiotics. Let your children play in the mud. Let your mouth maintain its own bacterial balance instead of nuking it with mouthwash every morning. These are small changes, but they matter more than most people realise.

And step four, the one that underpins everything else, is to address the insulin. Because as long as your insulin is chronically elevated, the metabolic environment inside your body will continue to promote inflammation, damage your gut lining, and undermine the very ecosystem that is trying to protect you.

• • •

The Defence You Did Not Know You Had

We spend billions on pharmaceuticals to fight infection, reduce inflammation, manage allergies and suppress autoimmune diseases. But yet we have, built into our biology, a defence system of breathtaking sophistication. One hundred trillion microbial partners, trained over millions of years of evolution, working in concert with an immune system that is capable of extraordinary precision when it is properly supported.

And we have been systematically dismantling it. Big food corporates stripped the fibre from our food because it made us consume more foods, making them bigger profits. We flooded ourselves with sugar that feeds the wrong bacteria and drives insulin resistance. We sanitised our environments until the beneficial microbes had nowhere left to live. And then we wondered why allergies exploded, why autoimmune diseases tripled, and why our children are sicker than any generation before them.

The solution is not complicated. It is not expensive. It does not require a prescription. It requires fibre, variety, and a willingness to stop doing the things that are destroying the ecosystem inside you.

80% of your immune system lives in your gut. What are you feeding it?

CHAPTER TEN

What the Government Are Getting Wrong

• • •

The late Bishop Desmond Tutu once said something that I come back to again and again. He said: there comes a point where we need to stop just pulling people out of the river. We must go upstream and find out why they are falling in.

That is exactly what is happening with chronic disease in this country. The NHS is standing at the bottom of the river, heroically pulling people out as fast as it can. But the river is getting wider and faster every year. More people are falling in than can be rescued. And nobody in a position of authority is willing to walk upstream and ask the obvious question: what is pushing them in?

This chapter is about that question. And the answers are uncomfortable.

I spend time in the House of Lords. I sit in the same rooms as the people who shape health policy in this country. I have looked them in the eye and told them what you are about to read. Some listened. Most did not. What follows is not the view of an outsider shouting from the sidelines. It is what I have seen, first-hand, from inside a system that knows it is broken and as of yet lacks the courage to fix it.

• • •

The Eatwell Guide

In the UK, the official dietary advice is built around a framework called the Eatwell Guide. It tells the public what a healthy plate should look like. And if you follow it, roughly half of your daily calories will come from starchy carbohydrates: bread, rice, pasta, potatoes and cereals. You are told to eat plenty of fruit and vegetables, which sounds sensible until you realise that fruit juice is included in that category. You are told to choose low-fat dairy. You are told to limit saturated fat.

Isabella's KetoSAge study tested exactly what happens when healthy people follow these guidelines. The participants were not asked to eat junk food. They were simply asked to increase their carbohydrate intake to match the government recommendations. They ate plenty of fruit. They avoided seed oils. They followed the official advice to the letter.

In just three weeks, their GLP-1 levels dropped by a factor of 2.4. Not a gentle decline. A collapse. Their fasting insulin rose. Their IGF-1 increased. Their liver enzymes shifted into the danger zone. Their mood changed. Their hunger returned with a vengeance, waking them up with stomach growls by day seven or eight.

Three weeks. That is all it took for the government's own recommended diet to produce measurable metabolic damage in women who had previously been in excellent health:

"Get rid of the UK standard Eatwell Guide. The UK food guidelines are wrong. They are highly flawed and they are not doing any favours for anyone. They are harming our children. They are causing more disease in patients in the NHS already, and they are actually harming our military. And very arguably they are harming our population growth as well."

When Isabella said that she was not being dramatic. She was reading her own data.

The Low-Fat Disaster

To understand how we ended up here, you need to go back to the middle of the twentieth century. In the 1950s, heart disease was rising rapidly in the Western world, and the scientific community was desperate to find a cause. One theory gained enormous traction: that saturated fat raised cholesterol, and that cholesterol caused heart disease. Eat less fat, the theory went, and you would have fewer heart attacks.

And that is exactly what happened. From the late 1970s onwards, the food supply was transformed. Low-fat products flooded the shelves, every one of them loaded with sugar to make up for the lost flavour. Cereals became sweeter. Yoghurts became desserts. Fruit juice was repositioned as a health food. The nation dutifully followed the government's advice, switched to low-fat everything, and proceeded to get fatter and sicker than ever before.

Diabetes rates have doubled in twenty years. One in two children born today will be diagnosed with cancer at some point in their lives. The NHS is teetering on the brink of collapse under the weight of chronic disease. And the dietary advice that was supposed to fix all of this has been in place for decades. It is not working. It has never worked. And the data has been telling us that for a very long time.

• • •

Ten Companies, One Strategy

But the low-fat deception was only half the story. The other half, and in some ways the more damaging half, is what happened when the food industry realised what fibre was costing them.

A mere ten corporate giants control the majority of what ends up on our plates. Ten companies. Ten boardrooms. Ten groups of food scientists who all arrived at the same conclusion: remove the fibre, and people eat more. It is that simple. Fibre reduces shelf life. It changes texture. It makes processing more complex. But the real problem, from a profit perspective, is that fibre makes you feel full. It slows down the sugar hit. It lowers the bliss point. And a lower bliss point means fewer repeat purchases. So over the course of a few decades, fibre was quietly and systematically stripped from the food supply.

Bread was refined until the fibre was gone. Cereals were processed until what remained was essentially sugar-flavoured dust. Fruit was turned into juice, which strips out the fibre entirely and leaves nothing but liquid sugar. This was not an accident. It was a commercial decision, made by corporations that understood exactly what they were doing. Because fibre is the one thing that stands between the sugar in your food and the insulin spike in your blood. Remove the fibre, and the sugar hits your bloodstream faster. The exact thing that is a disaster for your health, your insulin surges, is the very tool these corporations use to sell more product.

And the government has allowed this monopoly to take hold unchallenged. Ten boardrooms control what an entire nation eats, and not a single regulator has questioned whether that concentration of power might be part of the problem. Ten boardrooms getting rich while the rest of us get sick. That is not a free market. It is a failure of oversight on an epic scale.

If your meal comes dressed in a vibrant box, packet or tin, especially if it is making health claims on the label, you should approach it with extreme caution. Because the very companies selling you the food are the same companies that stripped out the ingredient that would have protected you from it.

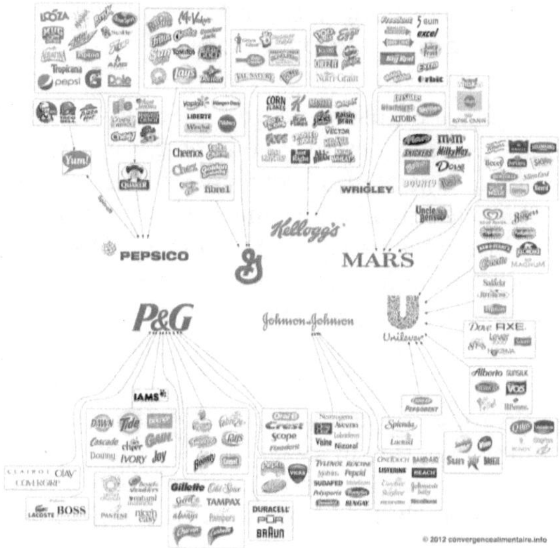

• • •

The GLP-1 Catch-22

This brings us to what I consider one of the most extraordinary contradictions in modern public health.

The government recommends a high-carbohydrate diet through the Eatwell Guide. Isabella's research has shown that a high-carbohydrate diet suppresses the body's natural production of GLP-1, the hormone that controls appetite and helps regulate blood sugar. When your GLP-1 production crashes, you become hungrier. You eat more. You gain weight. You develop insulin resistance. And eventually, you end up in your GP's surgery being told you need to lose weight.

And what does the government then fund your doctor to prescribe? A GLP-1 receptor agonist. An injection that replaces the very hormone that the government's own dietary guidelines suppressed in the first place.

Read that again, because it is worth letting it sink in. The official dietary advice destroys your body's natural appetite control system. And then the official medical response is to sell you a pharmaceutical replacement for the system they just destroyed. The guidelines cause the problem. The prescription manages the symptom. And nobody in the middle thinks to ask whether perhaps the guidelines themselves might be the issue.

And what do I mean when I say the government funds your GP to recommend a weight loss jab. At the time of writing this book, your GP can earn an extra £3,000 a year if he or she is prescribing the weight loss drugs to patients! How backwards is that?

It gets worse. When people come off the GLP-1 injections, as many eventually do, their natural GLP-1 production is still suppressed because they are still eating the high-carbohydrate diet they were told to follow. The hunger comes roaring back. The weight piles on, often faster than before. The patient feels like a failure. They blame themselves. They assume they lack willpower. But it was never about willpower. It was about biology that was sabotaged by the very advice they were given.

• • •

The Reference Ranges Nobody Questions

There is another way that the system fails people, and it is more subtle but just as damaging. It is the reference ranges that doctors use to assess your health.

When your GP sends you for a blood test, the results come back with a range marked as normal. If your number falls within that range, you are told you are fine. The problem is that those ranges were established using population studies. They represent what is average in the population. And when the population is overwhelmingly metabolically unhealthy, what is average drifts upwards until it no longer has any relationship with what is actually healthy.

Isabella identified this specifically with liver function tests. In her KetoSAge study, the participants' liver enzymes were healthy at levels under 14. The UK reference range for women goes up to 30. When men and women are pooled together, the range stretches as high as 50. That means a doctor can look at a liver enzyme level of 25, which in Isabella's data would indicate fatty liver disease, and tell the patient everything is normal.

Sixty or seventy years ago, children never had fatty liver disease. Today, one in four children have it. But if their liver enzymes fall within the reference range, they are told there is nothing wrong. The reference range has become a comfort blanket that obscures the damage until it is too late to prevent it.

The same problem applies to fasting insulin. Most GPs do not test fasting insulin at all. They test blood glucose and HbA1c. And as we discussed in the diabetes chapter, your blood sugar can remain perfectly normal for ten, fifteen, even twenty years while your insulin is sky-high and doing damage to every organ in your body. By the time your blood sugar finally rises enough to trigger a diagnosis, the insulin resistance has been running silently for decades. My dad's gout, blood pressure and erectile dysfunction were all warning signals that nobody connected because nobody measured the one thing that would have explained them all.

• • •

Follow the Money

At this point you might be asking the obvious question. If the science is this clear, why has nothing changed? Why are the guidelines still built around a high-carbohydrate model that the evidence has been contradicting for years?

I wish I could give you an innocent explanation. I wish I could tell you it is just bureaucratic inertia or honest disagreement among scientists. But I do not believe that is the full picture.

The food industry is enormous. The breakfast cereal market alone in the UK is worth two and a half billion pounds a year. Kellogg's products grace 17.5 million breakfast tables every morning. The soft drinks industry, the snack industry, the ready meal industry, the fruit juice industry, all of them are built on cheap carbohydrates, refined sugars and products that have had their fibre stripped away. If the government turned around tomorrow and told the public to eat fewer carbohydrates and more fat, to skip the orange juice and the cereal and the low-fat yoghurt, the financial consequences for those industries would be devastating.

And then there is the pharmaceutical industry. Insulin resistance and the diseases it causes are, collectively, the most profitable medical conditions on earth. Diabetes medication. Cholesterol-lowering statins. Blood pressure drugs. GLP-1 injections that cost hundreds of pounds a month. Cancer treatments. Alzheimer's medication. Every branch of the tree represents a revenue stream. If people prevented these diseases through diet, those revenue streams would dry up.

I mean, who can make money out of telling you to eat less, try intermittent fasting, and sleep more? These are all anti-money-making solutions. I wrote in *The Fibre First Diet* that this is an inconvenient truth for the bigwigs of the food and pharmaceutical industries. They are not about to let their multibillion-pound profits vanish. And as long as those industries have influence over the guidelines, over the research funding, and over the advice that doctors are trained to give, the guidelines will continue to protect the profits rather than the people.

• • •

The NHS Is Not the Villain

I want to be clear about something. I am not attacking the NHS. The doctors, nurses and healthcare workers in this country are extraordinary people doing extraordinary work under impossible pressure. The NHS was built to deal with acute illness, infections, injuries and emergencies, and it does that brilliantly.

But the NHS was never designed to manage an epidemic of chronic lifestyle disease. It was built for a world where people got sick from infections and accidents, not from the food they were told to eat. And it is now drowning under the weight of conditions that, in the majority of cases, could have been prevented or reversed if the dietary advice had been right from the beginning.

Imagine the NHS saving billions while preventing heart disease, cancer, diabetes, strokes and Alzheimer's, all by harnessing nutrition as medicine rather than depending solely on pharmaceuticals. That is not a fantasy once you realise it's the insulin. It is what the science says is possible. But it requires a fundamental shift in the advice that is given to the public. And that shift threatens too many powerful interests for it to happen easily.

CHAPTER ELEVEN

The Weight Loss Jab

• • •

Let me say something right at the start of this chapter. If you are on a GLP-1 injection, whether that is Ozempic, Wegovy, Mounjaro, Zepbound or Saxenda, I am not here to judge you. If the injection has helped you lose weight and feel better about yourself, I am genuinely glad. You made a decision with the information you had, and nobody should criticise you for that. And I would like to state for the record, that I am not anti-jab. It definitely has its place and has undoubtedly helped kick start recovery for some people.

But you deserve the full picture. And most people on these injections were never given it.

• • •

What the Injection Actually Does

GLP-1 stands for glucagon-like peptide-1. It is a hormone your body makes naturally, every time you eat real food. When food hits specialised cells in your gut called L-cells, they release GLP-1 into your bloodstream. It does two important things. First, it tells your brain you are full. Stop eating. Enough. Second, it slows down how quickly food moves through your stomach, so you stay satisfied for longer.

That is all perfectly natural and healthy. The human body has been doing it for millions of years.

The injection is a pharmaceutical GLP-1 receptor agonist, meaning a synthetic molecule designed to activate the same receptor as your body's natural GLP-1, but far more powerfully. It is not the same as the GLP-1 your body produces. It mimics the signal, but it dials it up to a level far beyond anything your body would ever create on its own.

Professor Ben Bikman, whose PhD lab was one of the first in the United States funded to study these gut hormones, described the early versions as relatively modest. He explains how the original drug was designed to treat type 2 diabetes at a low dose, and it worked well for that. It inhibited glucagon, brought blood sugar down, and as a side effect, people ate a little less.

Then the pharmaceutical industry spotted an opportunity. They took the same molecule, increased the dose four or five times, gave it a new name and a new patent, and suddenly it was no longer a diabetes drug. It was a weight loss drug. And the main mechanism, stripped of all the marketing language, is essentially a slowing of the intestines to such a degree that food sits in your stomach for more than twenty-four hours. When people say the food noise goes away, what they really mean is that they feel too full and too nauseous to want to eat.

• • •

The Thermostat and the Boiler

There is a way of thinking about this that I find helpful. Imagine your central heating is broken. The thermostat does not work, so the house is always cold. The injection is like hiring someone to stand next to the boiler all day, manually turning it on and off. The house stays warm. But the thermostat is still broken. The moment that person leaves, the house goes cold again.

That is what the injection does. It overrides your appetite signals. It makes you eat less by overwhelming one hormone.

But it does nothing about the other hormone that matters, which is insulin. The fat storage switch is still stuck. The insulin resistance that made you gain weight in the first place has not been addressed. And the moment you stop the injection, you have lost your appetite control and you have never fixed the underlying metabolic problem.

This is not speculation. A major Oxford University study published in the BMJ in January 2026 tracked over 9,000 adults and found that people on the weight loss injections regain weight at roughly 0.8 kilograms per month after stopping. That is nearly two pounds a month. At that rate, you are back to your starting weight in about eighteen months.

The Oxford team found something even more telling. They compared people who lost weight through injections with people who lost weight through diet and exercise. The drug group regained weight faster. Significantly faster. Because they never had to learn the skills to manage their appetite or their insulin. The thermostat was still broken.

• • •

The Muscle Problem

Here is something that troubles me deeply, and it should trouble you too if you're on the jab. Up to 40% of the weight you lose on these injections is not fat. It is muscle. Lean tissue. The stuff that keeps your metabolism running, that keeps you strong, that helps with insulin sensitivity.

When the weight comes back, and the data tells us that for most people it does, it comes back as fat. So, you can end up at the same weight you started at, but with more fat, less muscle, and worse insulin resistance than before you began. You are metabolically worse off than if you had never taken the injection at all.

Ben Bikman explained this in terms of metabolic rate. Normally, when a person loses weight, their metabolic rate drops a little. When they regain, the metabolic rate comes back up. It is not perfect, it lags slightly, but the system broadly works. However, when weight loss is dramatic and driven by eating less rather than eating right, the metabolic rate can uncouple from body weight entirely. A major meta-analysis looked at every available study comparing low-carb and high-carb weight loss. Both groups lost weight. But the high-carb, calorie-restricted group saw a substantial drop in their base metabolic rate. The low-carb group did not. Their metabolic rate stayed essentially the same.

That distinction matters enormously. If you lose weight through an injection that simply makes you eat less, without changing what you eat, you risk the same metabolic uncoupling. Your metabolism slows. And when you stop the injection and the hunger returns, you are fighting a slower engine with a broken thermostat. The weight comes back faster than it left.

• • •

What Nobody Told You About the Side Effects

The research I submitted to the House of Lords included some numbers that I believe every person considering these injections should see. A study of over 162,000 patients found a 195% higher risk of major depression.

Ben told me something during our interviews that stayed with me. He said it is not just that people feel depressed in the clinical sense. It is more that life becomes flat. Everything that used to bring them joy, hiking, intimacy, hobbies, passions, just fades. The word he used was apathy. The injection does not just suppress the desire to eat. It suppresses desire full stop. Because GLP-1 receptors are not just in your gut. They are in your brain, affecting dopamine and pleasure. They are in your heart. They are in your pancreas. When you flood all of those receptors with a synthetic agonist at supraphysiological levels, you do not just lose your appetite. You lose something harder to define:

"When you inject a GLP-1 receptor agonist, that becomes the only source of GLP-1 signalling in your body. Your own natural production shuts down. And the side effects we are seeing, the depression, the anxiety, the bone and muscle loss, these are not anomalies. They are the predictable consequences of replacing a finely tuned biological system with a pharmaceutical sledgehammer."

Isabella does not mince her words. And the data supports every one of them.

• • •

The Two-Hormone Problem

This is the critical point that almost everyone misses, including many of the doctors prescribing these drugs. Weight regulation is not a one-hormone problem. It is a two-hormone problem. You need to address both insulin and GLP-1.

1. Insulin as we have already seen is the fat storage hormone. When it is chronically elevated, your body cannot burn its own fat. It is locked away. You could eat almost nothing and still struggle to lose weight because insulin is holding the door shut. That is what insulin resistance does. The injection does absolutely nothing to address it.

2. GLP-1 is an appetite hormone. When it is working properly, you feel satisfied after eating. You do not experience constant hunger or cravings. Your body produces it naturally when you eat real food, particularly when fibre hits those L-cells in your gut.

The injection addresses one hormone by flooding it artificially, while completely ignoring the other. It makes you eat less, but it does not fix the metabolic machinery that made you gain weight. It suppresses the symptom without treating the cause. And that is why the weight comes back.

What if you addressed both? What if you could boost your natural GLP-1 production so your appetite was under control, and bring your insulin down so your body could actually burn fat? That is not a hypothetical. That is what happens when you change the way you eat. The weight does not just come off. It stays off. Because you have fixed the thermostat, not just hired someone to stand next to the boiler.

• • •

Your Body Already Knows How to Do This

Your body already makes GLP-1. It has been doing it since the day you were born. The problem is that most people are not producing enough of it, because the modern diet has suppressed it. As we discussed in the previous chapter, the government's own dietary guidelines push a high-carbohydrate diet that crashes your natural GLP-1 production. Isabella's KetoSAge study showed a 2.4-fold decrease with participants in just three weeks.

But the reverse is also true. When you eat in a way that keeps insulin low, your body starts making its own GLP-1 again. Fibre directly stimulates the L-cells of the small intestine to produce GLP-1. Protein increases it. Certain fats increase it. Even specific foods and supplements can boost production by 40 to 50%.

Ben Bikman put it beautifully. He said that GLP-1 is undoubtedly a metabolic advantage. We want it. But we want our own GLP-1, produced by our own bodies, at levels that our biology is designed to handle. Not a synthetic version injected at four or five times the natural concentration, paralysing the gut and flattening the joy out of life.

• • •

A Better Path for Those on the Injection

If you are currently on a GLP-1 injection and you want to come off it safely, Ben has a clear recommendation based on his research. And it does not involve stopping the drug overnight.

The first step is to change what you eat while you are still on the injection. Move towards a diet that is low in carbohydrates, high in quality fats and proteins. This does several things at once. It starts to lower your insulin. It begins to restore your body's natural GLP-1 production. And critically, it preserves your muscle mass, which the injection alone is stripping away.

As your natural hormone production recovers, Ben suggests a microdosing approach, gradually reducing the dose of the injection rather than stopping it abruptly. Your body needs time to pick up the slack. Think of it as a handover. The injection has been doing the work. Now you are teaching your body to do the work again. You reduce the dose as your own systems come back online.

This is not something you should do without your GP's knowledge and support. That is non-negotiable. But it is something that thousands of people have already done successfully, and the science behind it is robust. Isabella says:

"If someone is on a GLP-1 agonist and they also transition to a well-formulated ketogenic diet, they can often reduce to a

much lower dose. We call it microdosing. The combination works better at a lower dose with fewer side effects, and it gives the body time to restore its own production. The goal is always to get the person to a place where their own biology is doing the job the injection was hired to do."

• • •

The Real Scandal

I want you to hold two things in your mind at once. First, the government recommends a diet that suppresses your body's natural GLP-1 production. Second, the government then funds your doctor to prescribe an injection that replaces the very hormone their dietary advice destroyed. The guidelines cause the problem. The prescription manages the symptom. And the patient is left believing it is their own fault that they cannot control their weight.

It is not their fault. It was never their fault. The system failed them. The dietary advice failed them. And then when the injection inevitably stops working or becomes intolerable, they are left heavier, weaker, and more metabolically damaged than before.

That is not healthcare. That is a treadmill. And the only people who benefit from it are the pharmaceutical companies selling the drug and the food companies selling the diet that made the drug necessary in the first place.

There is a better way. Your body already has the machinery to regulate your weight, control your appetite, and keep you healthy. It just needs the right fuel. Everything you need to know about providing that fuel is in the chapters that follow.

Life Beyond the Jab

If you have read this far, you understand something that most people never get told. You understand the tree. You understand how insulin resistance sits at the root of obesity, type 2 diabetes, cancer, heart disease, Alzheimer's, and dozens of other conditions that are treated as separate illnesses but share the same underlying cause. You understand how the government's own dietary guidelines made the problem worse, and how the pharmaceutical industry turned the consequences into a product.

The question is: what do you do about it?

When I wrote the House of Lords paper with Isabella and Ben, and when Clubwell built the GLMe-1 programme, a seven-day online video course designed to help people transitioning off the weight loss drugs, we were very clear about one thing: there is no single approach that works for everyone.

Some people love their bread. Some love pasta. Others love rice. Asking them to give up carbohydrates entirely is asking them to fight a battle on two fronts, against their appetite and against their relationship with food. For some people, that is too much, especially at the start.

So, we designed three pathways, all leading to the same destination: a body that regulates its own weight without pharmaceutical help.

The first pathway is fibre-forward. You keep some of your carbohydrates, but you add 30 grams of fibre a day and you change the order in which you eat. Fibre first, then protein, then carbohydrates. This stimulates your L-cells, boosts your natural GLP-1, and blunts the blood sugar spike from the carbohydrates that follow. It is the gentlest approach, and it works particularly well for people who are not ready to give up their favourite foods.

The second pathway is the insulin approach. You dramatically reduce carbohydrates by following a ketogenic style diet, bringing insulin down and switching your body into fat-burning mode. This is faster. The KetoSAge research showed measurable improvements within weeks. And because low insulin also doubles GLP-1 production, you get both hormones working in your favour from the same dietary change.

The third pathway is the hybrid. You combine both levers. Fibre to stimulate GLP-1 from the gut, carbohydrate reduction to bring insulin down, and the lifestyle tools we discuss in our GLMe-1 course stacked on top.

None of these pathways requires perfection. They are starting points. You can move between them. You can start gentle and build. The tools work however you combine them.

If you are currently on a GLP-1 injection, you do not have to stop tomorrow. You may not need to stop at all. But if and when you are ready, there is a safe, gradual way to transition. It starts with building the foundation while you are still on the injection. Changing what you eat. Introducing fibre. Reducing carbohydrates. Getting the lifestyle pieces in place. Then, with your GP's knowledge and support, gradually reducing the dose as your body's own systems come back online.

This is not medical advice, and any changes to your medication must be made with your GP. But it is a conversation worth having. And it is a conversation you can walk into informed, with data, with a plan, and with an understanding of the science that most patients are never given.

• • •

GLMe-1: Life Beyond the Weight Loss Jabs

Everything I have described in this chapter, the two-hormone framework, the three pathways, the natural GLP-1 toolkit, the transition plan, the microdosing concept, is covered in detail in my seven-day programme, *GLMe-1: Life Beyond the Weight Loss Jabs*. It is a complete, step-by-step online video course that takes you from understanding the science to having a practical daily protocol that works with your biology instead of against it.

Day by day, I walk you through insulin and why it matters, how to boost your natural GLP-1 through fibre, food, supplements, movement and sleep, the three pathways so you can choose the approach that fits your life, the transition plan for reducing or stopping the injection safely, and what the first 30 days of life after the jab actually look like.

It is the programme I wish had existed when I was obese. And it is the programme that Clubwell built because we believe nobody should have to choose between a drug that makes them miserable and a weight they cannot control.

If you are interested, you can find it at clubwell.com. But whether you take the programme or not, the science in this book stands on its own. You now understand the tree. You understand the roots. And you understand that there is a path through the branches that does not require a pharmaceutical company to hold your hand.

• • •

A Note on the Clubwell App

Throughout this book I have deliberately kept product mentions to a minimum. This is a science book, not a sales pitch. But it would be dishonest of me not to mention the tool we built specifically to support everything in this chapter.

The totally free Clubwell app includes a food diary that tracks your nutritional intake and blood measurements, a journal for monitoring hunger, energy and mood, lifestyle tracking for sleep and movement, and access to the community of people walking the same path. If you are transitioning off the injection, the app gives you data you can take to your GP. If you are simply trying to eat better, it keeps you accountable.

You do not need the app to benefit from this book. Everything in these pages works with nothing more than the food on your plate. But if you want the structure and the support, it is there and it's totally free. That is all I will say about it.

CHAPTER TWELVE

What Happens When You Eat

• • •

For years, people have asked me to explain in simple terms what actually happens inside our bodies when we eat. Not the vague version. Not the version that talks about calories in and calories out. The real version. The biological truth of what happens to the food on your plate from the moment it enters your mouth to the moment it either fuels you or harms you.

And the story starts earlier than you think. There are two separate responses happening through completely different pathways. The moment sugar hits your tongue, your taste buds send a signal directly to your brain's reward centre, and dopamine is released almost instantly. This happens before a single molecule of sugar has been swallowed, let alone absorbed. Your pancreas even starts releasing a small amount of insulin just from tasting sweetness, before any sugar reaches your bloodstream. Then, about 15 to 30 minutes later, when glucose has been absorbed through the small intestine, passed through the liver, and reached the general bloodstream, the second response kicks in. This is the metabolic one. The real glucose arriving in your blood. This chapter is about that second response. The full mechanical story of what happens once food leaves your mouth.

But before we get going, it's important to know that virtually everything you eat, once digested, is broken down into just three types of molecules, carbohydrates (which become sugar), fats (lipids), and proteins (amino acids). We call these macronutrients.

If your food once had a face (think meat, fish) or came from something that once had a face (think eggs, cheese, yoghurt), it's primarily made up of fats and proteins. If it grew rooted in the ground (think vegetables, grains, fruits), it's mainly carbohydrates with some protein. Simple as that.

It also helps to understand what each of these three macronutrients is actually for, because they do very different jobs.

Carbohydrates are pure fuel. Your body breaks them down into glucose, and glucose has one primary purpose: to be burned for energy. It is the quick-access fuel, the kindling on the fire. There is no minimum human requirement for carbohydrates. Zero. Your body needs essential fatty acids. It needs essential amino acids. But there is no such thing as an essential carbohydrate. Every gram of glucose your body needs, it can manufacture itself through gluconeogenesis.

Fats are dual-purpose. They can be burned for energy, particularly when insulin is low, but they are also essential building materials. Every cell membrane in your body is made from fat. Your brain is roughly 60% fat. Without it, your body cannot maintain its own structure.

Protein is different again. Protein is primarily a builder, not a fuel. When you eat protein, your digestive system breaks it down into amino acids, small molecules that are reassembled into muscle, bone, skin, enzymes, hormones, and immune cells. There are twenty amino acids in total, and nine of them are called essential because your body cannot make them. You have to eat them. This is why protein from animal sources, meat, fish, eggs, and dairy, is considered complete: it contains all nine essential amino acids in the right proportions. Most plant proteins are missing one or more. Your body can burn protein for energy if it has to, but that is a last resort, like burning the furniture to heat the house. Protein's real job is to build and repair you.

What now follows may be the most important few pages in this book. We are going to walk through the entire metabolic process step by step, first for what happens universally to all food, and then for the two very different outcomes depending on a single factor: how much insulin is in your blood.

Step 1: The Stomach

When food hits your stomach, these three macronutrients go on very different journeys. Carbohydrates have a head start because salivary amylase in your mouth has already begun breaking starches into simpler sugars while you were still chewing. Protein gets worked on next, with pepsin, a powerful enzyme released by your stomach lining, breaking it down into smaller chains called peptides. Fat barely gets touched. It floats on top of everything else and waits.

Nothing enters your bloodstream from the stomach. Not a single molecule of protein, fat, or carbohydrate. The stomach is purely a breakdown and holding tank. It churns everything into a paste called chyme, then releases it in controlled bursts through a valve called the pyloric sphincter (located inside the pylorus) into the duodenum, the first section of the small intestine. That is where absorption begins. The only two exceptions are alcohol and certain medications like aspirin, which are small enough to pass directly through the stomach wall. Glucose, despite being one of the smallest sugar molecules in nature, just six carbon atoms, six oxygen atoms, and twelve hydrogen atoms, still cannot get through. Even something that tiny has to wait its turn and travel to the small intestine before it enters your blood.

Here is the first advantage of a low-carb meal: fat slows the pylorus down. The more fat in the meal, the more slowly the stomach releases its contents through the pyloric sphincter into the small intestine. So, in a low-carb meal, which is typically higher in fat and protein, the glucose trickle into the duodenum is slower and steadier from the very start.

Step 2: The Small Intestine

As the chyme passes through the pylorus and enters the duodenum, two things happen almost immediately. The pancreas releases digestive enzymes to finish breaking down all three macronutrients. And the gallbladder squirts bile into the mix, which is essential for breaking fat into tiny droplets small enough to be absorbed.

The inside of your small intestine is not smooth. It is covered in millions of tiny finger-like projections called villi, and each one is covered in even smaller projections called microvilli. If you could flatten them all out, the total surface area would be roughly the size of a tennis court. Inside each villus sit two things side by side: a network of tiny blood capillaries, and a small lymphatic vessel called a lacteal. Glucose and amino acids are absorbed into the capillaries. Fat is absorbed into the lacteals. The two different pipelines we are about to discuss start right here, at the microscopic level, inside each tiny finger of tissue.

Those thousands of capillaries merge into larger and larger veins, all eventually combining into one single blood vessel called the portal vein, which delivers the glucose and amino acids directly to the liver.

The lacteals, meanwhile, feed into the lymphatic system, carrying the fat on a completely separate journey that bypasses the liver altogether.

But here is what matters most: the pancreas is also watching. Special cells called beta cells are monitoring the glucose arriving in the small intestine. In a low-carb meal, not much glucose shows up. So, the pancreas releases only a small, measured amount of insulin. Just enough to handle what is there. No flood. No spike. A gentle, proportionate response.

The glucose is absorbed through the intestinal wall first. It is the smallest and simplest molecule, so it gets through fastest.

Protein, now broken down into amino acids, follows. Fat, broken into fatty acids, takes the longest because it has to be repackaged into chylomicrons, which are absorbed into the lacteals and sent into the lymphatic system rather than the portal vein.

In a low-carb meal, this whole process is calm and orderly. A small amount of glucose arrives, a small amount of insulin meets it, and nothing gets overwhelmed.

This is where fibre changes the game. Soluble fibre forms a gel in the stomach and small intestine that physically slows down the rate at which glucose is absorbed through the intestinal wall. A flatter spike means a gentler insulin response, which means no overshoot crash 90 minutes later, which means your brain does not scream for more food. Fibre does not block cravings by suppressing the pleasure response. Your tongue still tastes the sweetness and your brain still gets its dopamine. What fibre does is stop the crash that makes you chase the next hit. It breaks the cycle.

It is also worth noting that sweetness hitting the tongue signals the pancreas to release insulin in anticipation of what is coming. This is called the Cephalic Phase Insulin Response. It is why most artificial sweeteners still raise your insulin. They might not have calories, but elevated insulin, as you now know, locks your body in fat storage mode. People using sweeteners to lose weight are often sabotaging themselves without realising it.

Step 3: Two Different Pipelines

There is one more detail worth knowing, and it changes how you think about the fat you eat.

Every molecule of glucose and every amino acid from protein passes through the liver first, before it reaches the rest of your body. The liver acts as a gatekeeper, deciding what to store, what to process, and what to release.

As just mentioned, but worth repeating as it's so important to grasp, fat takes an entirely different route. Once absorbed, fatty acids are repackaged into transport molecules called chylomicrons and enter the lacteals, the tiny lymphatic vessels inside each villus. From there they travel through the lymphatic system, a separate network of vessels that bypasses the liver completely. They travel up through the body and empty into the bloodstream near your left shoulder via something called the thoracic duct. From there, fat circulates freely and can be picked up directly by your muscles, your fat cells, and your organs without the liver ever seeing it.

Two macronutrients go through the front door and get checked by security. Fat climbs in through the window.

And this is exactly why the quality of fat you eat matters so much. Protein and carbohydrate pass through the liver, which acts as a filter and can process, modify, or neutralise some of what comes through. Fat gets no such screening. Whatever fat you eat goes straight into your bloodstream and circulates around your body as is. If that fat is high quality, olive oil, butter, oily fish, coconut oil, avocado, your cells receive the building blocks they need. If it is seed oil, industrially extracted and chemically unstable, then that is what your cells, your membranes, and your mitochondria are being built from. There is no safety net. No gatekeeper. No second chance. What you eat is quite literally what you become.

All of this absorption happens in the small intestine. By the time what is left of your meal reaches the large intestine, virtually all the glucose, amino acids, and fatty acids have already been absorbed. The large intestine's job is different: it handles water absorption, electrolytes, and the fermentation of fibre by your gut bacteria, which is where those all-important short-chain fatty acids are produced. But the macronutrient story is over before it gets there.

The Fork in the Road

Everything you have just read happens the same way no matter what you eat. The stomach breaks it down. The small intestine absorbs it. Protein and carbohydrate go to the liver via the portal vein. Fat bypasses the liver and enters the bloodstream through the lymphatic system. That process is universal.

But from this point forward, your body takes one of two paths. Which one depends on a single thing: how much insulin is in your blood.

To be honest, if you have followed everything so far, you do not need this next section. But if you want to see the full picture laid out simply, here it is.

Glucose

LOW INSULIN (low-carb or ketogenic meal)

A small amount of glucose arrives in the bloodstream via the portal vein. The liver sits first in line and intercepts it, taking what it needs for its own energy and topping up its glycogen stores if they are not already full. The rest passes straight through into the general circulation, where it is available to any cell in the body that needs it. Your heart, lungs, muscles, brain, and kidneys can all pull glucose directly from the bloodstream. Insulin acts as the key, unlocking glucose transporters on the surface of these cells so the glucose can flow in.

In a low-carb meal, not much glucose shows up, so the pancreas releases only a small, measured dose of insulin. Just enough to open the doors that need opening. The cells that need immediate energy take what they need, and any surplus is stored as glycogen in the liver and muscles, the only two places your body can store it, up to a combined limit of around 400 to 500 grams. Blood sugar rises gently, then settles back down. The whole event is barely noticeable on a glucose monitor.

HIGH INSULIN (high-carb meal)

A large amount of glucose floods the portal vein. Remember, your body is designed to keep roughly one teaspoon of sugar in the bloodstream at any time. Everything your body is about to do is driven by one urgent priority: get that number back down to one teaspoon.

The liver sits first in line and intercepts what it can, burning some for immediate energy and filling its glycogen stores quickly. The excess passes straight through into the general bloodstream and blood sugar spikes, way beyond that one teaspoon. Every cell in your body that needs energy, your heart, lungs, muscles, brain, kidneys, can pull glucose directly from the bloodstream, and they do. But even with every cell taking what it needs, there is still too much.

The pancreas responds with a large surge of insulin. Insulin pushes glucose into muscle cells, where it is either burned for energy or stored as muscle glycogen. But there is a limit. Once both the liver and muscles have filled their glycogen tanks, roughly 400 to 500 grams combined, there is nowhere left for the glucose to go. And blood sugar is still above one teaspoon.

So, the liver starts converting the surplus glucose into fatty acids through *de novo lipogenesis*. It packages those fatty acids into triglycerides, wraps them in VLDL particles, and ships them back out into the bloodstream. The sugar you ate is now circulating as fat.

From there, insulin takes over. It activates lipoprotein lipase on the surface of your fat cells, which cracks open those VLDL parcels and pulls the fatty acids inside. Meanwhile, the smaller amount of glucose that insulin has pushed directly into fat cells is being used to build glycerol-3-phosphate, the scaffold needed to reassemble those fatty acids into triglycerides for long-term storage. The liver makes the fat. The fat cells build the frame to store it. Insulin orchestrates the entire operation.

All of this is your body doing whatever it takes to get blood sugar back down to one teaspoon. It is not a design flaw. It is an emergency response. The problem is when that emergency happens three, four, five times a day, meal after meal, day after day. Those cells begin to stop responding. The doors start to jam. That is insulin resistance.

The Liver

LOW INSULIN (low-carb or ketogenic meal)

The liver is calm. It has received a manageable amount of glucose via the portal vein, stored what it needs as glycogen, and let the rest pass through into the general circulation. Because insulin is low, the liver is free to do something remarkable: it starts pulling fatty acids from the bloodstream and converting them into ketones. This is the liver's secondary role, and it only kicks in when insulin is low enough to allow it. The liver becomes a ketone factory, producing clean, efficient fuel for your brain, heart, and kidneys.

It is worth noting that the liver itself does not burn the ketones it makes. It produces them and sends them out for other organs to use. It is a factory, not a customer.

HIGH INSULIN (high-carb meal)

The liver is overwhelmed. It has filled its glycogen stores and there is still glucose pouring in through the portal vein. With nowhere else to put it, the liver switches on *de novo lipogenesis*, converting the excess glucose into fatty acids. It packages those fatty acids into triglycerides, wraps them in VLDL particles, and ships them back out into the bloodstream. The liver has gone from being a gatekeeper to being a fat factory.

And here is the cruel part: the fat it is producing does not just get sent to your fat cells. Some of it stays behind. Triglycerides start to accumulate inside the liver itself. Do this often enough, meal after meal, year after year, and the result is non-alcoholic fatty liver disease, NAFLD. A condition that barely existed fifty years ago and is now one of the most common liver diseases in the Western world. It is not caused by drinking. It is caused by sugar.

Fat Cells

LOW INSULIN (low-carb or ketogenic meal)

Your fat cells are finally open for business, but in the opposite direction. With insulin low, hormone-sensitive lipase, an enzyme that works inside the fat cell, switches on and begins breaking down stored triglycerides into free fatty acids, releasing them back into the bloodstream where they can be picked up by muscles and other tissues for fuel.

At the same time, lipoprotein lipase, an enzyme that sits on the outer surface of your fat cells, quiets down, so fewer triglycerides are being pulled in from the blood. The entrance slows. The exit opens. You are burning stored body fat. This is what your body was designed to do between meals and overnight, but it can only happen when insulin is low enough to allow it.

HIGH INSULIN (high-carb meal)

Your fat cells are in full storage mode. Insulin activates lipoprotein lipase on the surface of your fat cells, which pulls triglycerides out of those VLDL parcels the liver just made and feeds the fatty acids inside. Meanwhile, the glucose being pushed into fat cells is converted into glycerol-3-phosphate, the scaffold needed to reassemble those fatty acids into triglycerides for long-term storage.

And the exit? Locked. Insulin suppresses hormone-sensitive lipase, so none of that stored fat can be broken down and released. Meanwhile, fat is arriving from the liver as VLDL triglycerides, pulled inside by lipoprotein lipase, while glucose is being pushed into the same fat cell and converted into the scaffolding needed to lock that fat into long-term storage. The raw materials are coming in from one direction and the construction crew from another, and nothing is getting out. This is the fat trap.

Muscles

LOW INSULIN (low-carb or ketogenic meal)

Your muscle cells are relaxed. They have received whatever small amount of glucose was available and burned it or stored it as glycogen. But because insulin is low, they have also switched on their ability to burn fatty acids directly through a process called beta-oxidation. Your muscles become fat-burning machines, pulling free fatty acids from the bloodstream and using them for fuel.

This is important because by burning fat directly, your muscles leave the ketones for the organs that need them most, the brain, the heart, and the kidneys. Your muscles are being selfless, taking the fat and passing the ketones upstairs.

Your muscles are also efficiently taking up amino acids from the protein you ate, using them for repair and growth. With fat providing the energy, protein can do what it is actually designed to do: build and maintain.

HIGH INSULIN (high-carb meal)

Your muscle cells are being bombarded with glucose. Insulin is forcing it through the door as fast as possible. The muscles burn what they can and store some as muscle glycogen, but there is a limit to how much they can hold. Once muscle glycogen is full, the excess glucose has to go somewhere else.

Meanwhile, because insulin is high, your muscles have switched off their ability to burn fat. They are locked into glucose-burning mode. This is called metabolic inflexibility – your body has lost the ability to switch between fuel sources – and it is one of the earliest signs that something is going wrong.

And there is a quieter casualty that most people never think about. As muscle cells become increasingly resistant to insulin over time, they also become less efficient at taking up amino acids from the protein you ate. Your muscles need those amino acids to repair and rebuild, but they are not getting the delivery they should. Over the years, this impairs your muscles' ability to maintain themselves, which is one of the reasons people with long-term insulin resistance tend to lose muscle mass, especially as they age. Any excess amino acids that the muscles fail to take up are sent back to the liver, which converts them into yet more glucose through *gluconeogenesis*, adding fuel to a fire that is already out of control.

The Brain

LOW INSULIN (low-carb or ketogenic meal)

The brain cannot burn fatty acids. They are too large to cross the blood-brain barrier. But it does not need to, because the liver is producing ketones, and ketones cross the blood-brain barrier with ease. Your brain switches from running on glucose to running on a mix of ketones and a small amount of glucose that the liver produces through *gluconeogenesis*.

Research suggests the brain runs efficiently on ketones, and many people report clearer thinking, better focus, and more stable mood when in ketosis. The brain is not starving. It is thriving on a cleaner fuel.

HIGH INSULIN (high-carb meal)

The brain is running entirely on glucose. When blood sugar spikes, the brain gets a burst of energy. When insulin then drives blood sugar back down, sometimes overshooting, the brain hits a wall. This is the post-meal fog, the afternoon slump, the inability to concentrate two hours after a sandwich. The brain is on a roller coaster (what I termed the carbocoaster), spiking and crashing with every meal.

Over time, chronic high insulin may also impair the brain's ability to use glucose efficiently. See previous chapter on cognitive decline and Alzheimer's disease.

The Heart

LOW INSULIN (low-carb or ketogenic meal)

The heart is in its happy place. It can burn fatty acids, glucose, or ketones, but research shows it runs most efficiently on ketones. In a low-insulin state, with ketones available and fatty acids circulating freely, the heart has access to its two preferred fuels. It is well supplied and working efficiently.

And here is something that often surprises people: when you eat more fat on a low-carb diet, your blood triglyceride levels typically go down, not up. That seems counterintuitive until you understand where blood triglycerides actually come from. They are not a direct reflection of the fat you eat. The triglycerides that show up on a fasting blood test are mainly the ones your liver made from sugar through *de novo lipogenesis*. In a low-insulin state, the liver is not doing that. It is making ketones instead. Less sugar in, fewer triglycerides out. The heart is bathing in clean fuel, not in fat manufactured from last night's pasta.

HIGH INSULIN (high-carb meal)

The heart is stuck burning glucose, a fuel it can use but does not prefer. It is also being exposed to high levels of circulating triglycerides from the liver's VLDL output, and high insulin is promoting inflammation in the arterial walls.

This is where a standard blood test tells an important story. High triglycerides on a fasting blood test are not caused by eating too much fat. They are a marker that your liver has been converting excess sugar into fat and shipping it out as VLDL. It is a sugar problem showing up on a fat measurement. Over time, this combination of high triglycerides and inflamed arterial walls contributes to atherosclerosis, the narrowing and hardening of arteries that leads to heart attacks and strokes.

The Kidney

LOW INSULIN (low-carb or ketogenic meal)

The kidneys, like the heart, are efficient ketone burners. They are well fuelled and under no particular stress. Blood pressure tends to be lower in a low-insulin state because insulin normally causes the kidneys to retain sodium and water. With insulin low, the kidneys release excess sodium and fluid naturally, which is why people often lose several pounds of water weight in the first week of a low-carb diet.

HIGH INSULIN (high-carb meal)

The kidneys are retaining sodium and water because insulin is telling them to hold on to it. This contributes to raised blood pressure. At the same time, elevated blood sugar is damaging the tiny blood vessels inside the kidneys, which over time leads to kidney disease, one of the most common complications of type 2 diabetes.

Red Blood Cells

LOW INSULIN (low-carb or ketogenic meal)

Red blood cells have no mitochondria, so they cannot burn fatty acids or ketones. They can only ever use glucose. But they do not need much, and your liver produces exactly what it requires through *gluconeogenesis*, making new glucose from amino acids. Even in deep ketosis, with zero carbohydrate intake, your red blood cells are never short of fuel. Your body has this covered.

HIGH INSULIN (high-carb meal)

Red blood cells are fine. They have more glucose than they could ever need. This is the one cell type that is not negatively affected by high insulin in the short term. But the excess glucose in the blood around them is causing damage everywhere else.

The End Result

LOW INSULIN (low-carb or ketogenic meal)

Your body is in balance. A small amount of glucose is handled calmly. Your liver is making ketones. Your fat stores are being unlocked and burned. Your muscles are running on fat. Your brain, heart, and kidneys are running on ketones. Your blood sugar is stable. Your blood pressure is healthy. Inflammation is low. You have steady energy from morning to night without crashes, cravings, or hunger. This is what your body was designed to do.

HIGH INSULIN (high-carb meal)

Your body is in crisis management. Too much glucose has arrived too fast. Your liver is converting the excess into fat. Your fat cells are stuffing themselves and locking the door. Your muscles are stuck in glucose-only mode. Your brain is on a sugar roller coaster. Your heart is bathing in triglycerides. Your kidneys are retaining water and your blood pressure is climbing.

And the worst part? You are hungry again two hours later, because the insulin crash that follows the spike drops your blood sugar below where it started, and your brain screams for more food. So, you eat again. I call it the carbocoaster and it's so damn important, I have included it in all of my health books to date!

CHAPTER THIRTEEN

The Ketogenic Diet

• • •

By now you understand the problem. Insulin resistance is the trunk of the tree, and almost every chronic disease we have discussed in this book grows from it. You also understand the solution in principle: get insulin down, and the body begins to heal itself. Fat stores open up. Inflammation quietens. The brain clears. The liver recovers.

The question many people begin asking once they understand what you have just read, is what's the ultimate way to drop my insulin level? If you are ready to go beyond simply reducing sugar and ultra-processed food, beyond eating fibre first, beyond cutting back, the most powerful tool I have come across in over a decade of research, personal experimentation, and conversations with some of the world's leading scientists is the ketogenic diet.

• • •

What a Ketogenic Diet Actually Is

A ketogenic diet is not complicated. You reduce your carbohydrate intake to below roughly 20 grams a day. That is not a lot. A single banana has about 27 grams. A slice of bread has around 15. So, we are talking about almost none.

When you remove carbohydrates to this degree, something remarkable happens. Your body, starved of its usual quick-burn fuel, has to find an alternative. It turns to fat. Your liver begins breaking down fatty acids from your fat stores and converting them into ketones. These ketones become your primary fuel source. Your brain runs on them. Your heart runs on them. Your muscles run on them. And as long as your carbohydrate intake stays low enough, this process continues day and night.

This is the state called ketosis. And it is not some extreme metabolic emergency. It is what your body was designed to do. As Dr Terry Wahls, who reversed her own progressive multiple sclerosis through diet, puts it: humans went into ketosis every winter for thousands of generations. It is the more natural state for our metabolism.

The general rule, confirmed by virtually every researcher I have spoken to, is that you need to keep total carbohydrate intake below 20 grams per day. Cross that threshold and you risk producing enough insulin to shut the whole process down. Keep your carbs below it, focus on quality fats, moderate protein intake, and your body will do the rest.

• • •

The Brain's Preferred Fuel

One of the most important things Ben Bikman taught me is that ketones are not some inferior backup fuel your body reluctantly switches to when glucose runs out. They are the brain's preferred fuel. Let me say that again, because it contradicts almost everything we have been taught. Ketones are the brain's preferred fuel.

As I mentioned earlier, if you take a person who has been fasting for 24 hours, their blood ketone levels might reach about one millimole per litre. At that point, the brain is already drawing roughly half its energy from ketones and only half from glucose. Now ask yourself: if the brain truly preferred glucose, why would it switch to ketones so eagerly the moment they become available? The brain does not reluctantly accept ketones. It reaches for them.

Ben points to newborn babies as further proof. A healthy baby enters a state of ketosis within hours of birth. Not mild ketosis either. A baby will reach a deeper state of ketosis in two hours than you or I would achieve in two days of fasting. The brain is growing faster in those early weeks than at any other point in life, and it is fuelled overwhelmingly by ketones. If ketones were an inferior fuel, nature would never have designed it this way.

This is also why people in ketosis so often report extraordinary mental clarity. I experienced it myself when I ran four marathons in five days completely fasted, and again when I cycled from Glasgow to Bristol over five days without eating. Every one of us on those experiments noticed the same thing: a sharpness of thought that felt almost superhuman. Ideas would flood my mind at night, and unlike the usual nocturnal musings that dissolve into nonsense by morning, the insights I scribbled down during ketosis were lucid, coherent, and genuinely profound.

• • •

Euketogenesis and Therapeutic Ketosis

For most of the last century, whenever doctors talked about ketosis it was in the context of danger. Diabetic ketoacidosis, a life-threatening condition in type 1 diabetes where ketone levels spiral out of control, cast a long shadow over the entire concept. Many doctors, even today, confuse the two. They hear the word ketones and immediately think of an emergency ward.

This confusion has held back the science for decades. Which is why a growing number of researchers, including Isabella

Cooper, are now pushing for clearer language. The term euketogenesis refers to the healthy, controlled production of ketones that occurs when a metabolically normal person restricts carbohydrates or fasts. "Eu" literally means "good" ketone creation and it is the body simply doing exactly what it evolved to do. You are said to be in euketogenesis when the level in your blood rises above 0.5 mmol/L.

Therapeutic ketosis takes it a step further. This is when ketosis is used deliberately as a medical intervention, whether for epilepsy, Alzheimer's, cancer, or metabolic disease. Or those strategically using it as a prevention tool for these same diseases and more. Therapeutic ketosis is generally considered to be around 2 mmol/L or approaching half of your blood glucose level.

The distinction matters. Euketogenesis is normal. Therapeutic ketosis is powerful medicine. Diabetic ketoacidosis is a medical emergency. They share a word, but they have almost nothing else in common.

• • •

What Happens in the Body

When you enter ketosis, the changes go far beyond weight loss. Ben's research has shown that when people are in ketosis, the metabolic rate of their belly fat triples. He and his team actually pulled biopsies of belly fat from people in ketosis and compared them to people who were not. The fat cells in the ketosis group were three times more active. They were burning, not just sitting there.

At the same time, ketones protect muscle tissue. This is one of the reasons a ketogenic diet is fundamentally different from simply starving yourself. When you cut calories without cutting carbohydrates, your body often cannibalises muscle for fuel. When you are in ketosis, the ketones effectively tell the body to leave the muscle alone and burn fat instead.

And there is another mechanism most people never hear about. When you are in ketosis, you are literally breathing out and urinating out calories. Every ketone molecule carries roughly the same caloric energy as a molecule of glucose. When your body produces more ketones than it immediately needs, the excess is expelled through your breath and your urine. You are losing energy without even trying. It is one of the reasons people in ketosis often lose weight faster than calorie calculations alone would predict.

• • •

Exogenous Ketones

The benefits of ketones are now so well established that companies have found ways to deliver them as a supplement. These are called exogenous ketones, meaning ketones produced outside the body, as opposed to endogenous ketones, which your liver makes internally.

They come in several forms. Ketone esters are the most potent. They deliver the actual ketone molecule, beta-hydroxybutyrate, directly into your bloodstream.

But here is a word of caution. Exogenous ketones are a tool, not a solution. They can be genuinely useful in specific situations: helping your brain through the difficult first week of carbohydrate restriction, giving a cognitive boost when you need one, or supporting someone with a neurological condition who struggles to maintain dietary ketosis.

What they cannot do is replace the diet itself. If you are drinking ketone supplements while still eating bread and pasta, your ketones might look fine on a monitor, and they may be helping your brain to perform better, but you still may have elevated insulin. The real power comes from your own body producing its own ketones, which only happens in a low insulin state. That is where the deep metabolic healing happens.

• • •

How to Know You Are in Ketosis

One of the things that makes the ketogenic diet unique among all diets is that you do not have to guess whether it is working. You can measure it.

There are three ways. A finger-prick blood meter gives you the most precise reading of beta-hydroxybutyrate in your blood. A breath monitor measures acetone, another ketone your body produces, and is painless and reusable. And urine strips, which cost next to nothing, give you a rough but useful indication, especially when you are starting out.

The numbers are straightforward. On a regular UK diet during the day, your ketone levels sit around zero to 0.1 millimoles per litre. When you wake up after an overnight fast, they might reach 0.3, which Ben actually considers the threshold of mild ketosis. That said, as I just mentioned, a more accepted range for euketogenesis is 0.5 to 2 millimoles per litre and above 2 millimoles you begin to enter therapeutic ketogenesis.

For context, diabetic ketoacidosis does not occur until levels hit around 25 millimoles per litre, a state that requires the near-total absence of insulin. It is not something a metabolically healthy person can accidentally stumble into.

If your monitor says you are in ketosis, your insulin is low. That is not a guess. It is biochemistry. And if your insulin is low, your body is burning fat, producing ketones, and allowing your cells to repair themselves. It is the most direct feedback loop any diet has ever offered.

• • •

The Ketogenic Transition

I will not pretend it is easy at first. Switching from a carbohydrate-heavy diet to a ketogenic one requires your body to build new metabolic machinery. You need to produce enzymes you have not needed in years, possibly decades. Nina Teicholz, the investigative journalist and nutrition researcher, described it on my podcast as having to develop all of these different enzymes to be able to run off fat. It is like restarting an engine that has been sitting idle in the garage.

For most people, the transition takes seven to 21 days. For those who have been eating a high-carbohydrate diet for a long time, it can stretch to six weeks. During that period, you might experience headaches, fatigue, irritability, or nausea. Some people call it keto flu. It is not a sign that something is wrong. It is a sign that something is changing. You are breaking a metabolic dependency that may have been running for your entire adult life.

The important thing is to get through it. Because once you are on the other side, the experience changes completely. Your energy stabilises. Your hunger fades, often dramatically. Your mental clarity sharpens. And you unlock access to your body's vast fat reserves, which hold anywhere between 40,000 and 200,000 calories of stored energy, compared to the meagre 2,000 to 2,500 calories of glycogen that a sugar-burner relies on.

• • •

A Word of Honesty

None of this means keto is right for everyone, or that it is easy to sustain. The compliance rate for strict ketogenic diets is notoriously low. Most studies that track participants beyond six months see a significant drop-off, and in real life, outside a clinical trial, the numbers are even worse. Social pressure, family meals, travel, and the sheer ubiquity of carbohydrates in modern food make long-term adherence difficult. That is not a failure of willpower. It is a reality of the world we live in. For some people, a less restrictive low-carbohydrate approach, one that still lowers insulin without requiring full ketosis, will be more sustainable and therefore more effective over a lifetime. If you try keto and find you cannot maintain it, that does not mean the science is wrong. It means a different degree of carbohydrate restriction might suit you better. The goal of this book is not to prescribe one single protocol. It is to get your insulin down, by whatever path you can actually walk.

• • •

A Note on Fibre

If you do go fully ketogenic, it is only fair for me to address something I have spent much of this book championing: fibre. As Isabella puts it, you do not need the antidote if you are not taking the poison. Fibre is the antidote to sugar. If you have removed the sugar, you might only need a small amount of fibre to feed your gut bacteria, and as yet, we do not have the science or data to prove even that is necessary.

That said, even when I am fasting or occasionally eating a carnivore diet, I still personally take a fibre supplement, because I do not want to risk the chance that we still need to support the microbiome, even when fibre is not needed as an antidote.

The Evidence

The research behind the ketogenic diet is no longer fringe. In 2022 alone, 604 peer-reviewed studies on the ketogenic diet were published in the PubMed database. By 2023, that number had risen to 726. Clinical trials have found in favour of the ketogenic diet for epilepsy, Alzheimer's disease, Parkinson's disease, cancer, weight loss, type 2 diabetes, PCOS, and migraine.

In fact, just about every metabolic marker gets better. Ben, Isabella, and I are all passionate about it, and the reason is simple: if you are in ketosis, it is proof that your insulin is low. You do not have to guess. You do not have to hope. You can measure it. And if this book has taught you anything, it should be this: getting insulin down is where the healing begins.

Glass of sugar-laden orange juice, anyone?

CHAPTER FOURTEEN

The Other Roots

• • •

By this point in the book, you understand something that most people never get told. Insulin resistance is driven, more than anything else, by what you eat. We have spent thirteen chapters examining how sugar, refined carbohydrates, ultra-processed products and stripped fibre combine to push your insulin through the roof and hold it there. And food is, without question, the biggest driver. If you fix nothing else but what you eat, you will transform your health.

But it is not the only driver. And this chapter is about the roots I have not yet dug into.

Go back to the *Tree of Afflictions* for a moment. We have spent most of this book looking at the branches, the diseases that grow from insulin resistance, and at the trunk itself. Now I want to take you underground, into the soil, where the roots feed the whole system.

If you divide those roots into two groups, the first group is the one we have been talking about all along. The dietary roots. Sugar. Foods stripped of fibre. Refined carbohydrates. Ultra-processed products. Seed oils. These are the roots that pump the most fuel into the trunk. They are the main supply line, and for most people, they are where the battle is won or lost.

But there are four other roots that also feed insulin resistance, and they do it whether or not your diet is perfect. A sedentary lifestyle. Chronic stress. Poor sleep. And certain medications. You could eat beautifully and still be feeding the tree through these other channels.

Before I go any further, I want to be honest about what this chapter is and what it is not. This is not a lifestyle manual. I am not going to give you a twenty-page sleep protocol or a detailed exercise programme. My book *The Fibre First Diet* covers over a thousand pages of practical how-to, and the free Clubwell app is built specifically to help you implement the plan, with recipes, community support, tracking tools and daily guidance. I did not want to duplicate all of that here.

What I do want to do is show you the science. Because once you understand why a sedentary afternoon or a bad night's sleep or chronic stress is feeding the same tree that a bowl of cornflakes feeds, your motivation to address them changes entirely. It stops being vague wellness advice and becomes specific, biological, and urgent.

Let us start with the one that affects almost everyone.

• • •

The Sitting Disease

We were not built to sit still. Every cell in your body was designed for movement. Your muscles, your bones, your cardiovascular system, your lymphatic drainage, your hormonal signalling, all of it was engineered over hundreds of thousands of years for a life spent on your feet, walking, lifting, carrying, climbing.

And yet here we are. Sitting at desks. Sitting in cars. Sitting on sofas. The average British adult now spends between nine and ten hours a day sedentary. That is more time than we spend sleeping. We have created a world so convenient that movement has become optional, and our bodies are paying the price in a currency most people never think about: insulin.

Here is the science, and it is worth understanding because it changes how you think about everything from your commute to your evening routine.

When you move, your muscles contract. When your muscles contract, they absorb glucose directly from your bloodstream and use it for energy. They do this through a protein we discussed earlier *GLUT4*, which acts like a doorman at a club, opening up the cell to let glucose in. Here is the remarkable part: active muscles do not need insulin to make this happen. During contraction, *GLUT4* moves to the surface of the muscle cell on its own. The glucose walks straight in. No insulin required.

The enzyme responsible for this is *AMPK*, your body's fuel gauge. When your muscles contract, *AMPK* switches on and triggers *GLUT*4 to move to the cell surface. It also tells your body to burn fat and build new mitochondria. When you sit all day, *AMPK* stays dormant.

Read that again if you need to. Your muscles, when they are working, can pull sugar out of your blood without any help from insulin whatsoever.

Now think about what happens when you sit for ten hours a day. Those *GLUT4* doors stay shut. The glucose builds up in your bloodstream. Your pancreas detects the rising sugar and does what it has been trained to do: it pumps out more insulin. But the muscles are not contracting, so they are not pulling glucose in. The insulin has to work harder, for longer, to achieve what a twenty-minute walk would have done effortlessly.

Do this every day for years, which is exactly what most of us do, and you get a slow, grinding increase in insulin resistance. Not because of what you ate, but because you did not move after you ate it. The engine was never turned on.

A South Korean study in 2019 found that people who sat for ten or more hours a day had significantly higher rates of hyperuricaemia (elevated uric acid, a marker closely linked to insulin resistance) than those who moved regularly. A separate analysis of over 226,000 people worldwide, published by the BBC, found that as few as 4,000 steps a day can measurably reduce the risk of premature death, and that every additional 1,000 steps cuts that risk by a further 15%, all the way up to 20,000 steps.

You do not need to run marathons. You do not need a gym membership. In fact, extreme exercise can sometimes do more harm than good. What you need is regular, consistent movement throughout the day. A walk after meals is one of the single most powerful things you can do for your insulin levels. Studies using continuous glucose monitors have shown that a gentle twenty to thirty-minute stroll after eating can dramatically flatten a blood sugar spike, sometimes by half. Your muscles wake up, *GLUT4* moves to the surface, and the glucose gets absorbed cleanly. No spike. No crash. No flood of insulin.

Dr Jeremy Morris proved this back in the 1950s, though nobody was paying much attention. He compared London bus drivers, who sat all day, with bus conductors, who climbed roughly 600 stairs per shift. The conductors had nearly 50% fewer heart attacks. He then studied postal workers and found the same pattern: those who walked and cycled had dramatically better cardiovascular health than those who stood behind counters. Dr Morris practised what he preached and lived to 99.

The message has not changed in seventy years. We just stopped listening.

If you have read the earlier chapters of this book, you understand that insulin resistance is the root system feeding almost every chronic disease we have discussed. Anything that reduces your body's reliance on insulin, anything that helps glucose get into your cells without insulin having to force the door open, is pulling up one of those roots. Movement does exactly that. It is free, it requires no prescription, and it works every single time you do it.

So, if you are reading this sitting down, here is a thought: finish the chapter on your feet.

• • •

The Sleep Debt

If someone told you there was a treatment that could reduce insulin resistance by 30%, curb your appetite, lower your cortisol, sharpen your brain, and strengthen your immune system, you would want to know how much it costs. The answer is nothing. It is sleep. And most of us are not getting enough of it.

Self-reported sleep duration has fallen by one and a half to two hours over the past four decades. In the 1960s, only 15% of young adults slept less than seven hours a night. Today that number is 37%. A recent survey found that nine in ten Britons say their life would improve if they got more sleep. They are right, and the reasons go far deeper than feeling tired.

Here is what happens to your insulin when you do not sleep.

Researchers at the University of Chicago split participants into two groups. One group was allowed to sleep normally. The other was restricted to four or five hours a night. After just one week of fragmented sleep, the deprived group showed a roughly 30% increase in insulin resistance. Not after months. Not after years. One week. Other studies have shown that the damage can begin after as little as two nights of poor rest.

Think about that in the context of everything else in this book. You could eat perfectly. You could avoid sugar, prioritise fibre, cut out ultra-processed food. But if you are sleeping five hours a night, your body is becoming insulin resistant anyway, because sleep deprivation triggers a hormonal cascade that undermines everything good you are doing with your fork.

The mechanism works like this. When you are sleep-deprived, your body produces more cortisol, the stress hormone. As we will see in the next section, cortisol tells your liver to release glucose into the bloodstream to prepare you for danger. But there is no danger. You are just tired. So now you have elevated blood sugar, and your pancreas responds with more insulin. Night after night, this becomes a pattern.

But cortisol is only half the story. Sleep deprivation also wrecks your hunger hormones. The Chicago researchers found that the sleep-deprived group woke up with elevated ghrelin (the hormone that tells you to eat) and suppressed leptin (the hormone that tells you to stop). Their bodies were sending a false famine signal. They were not actually hungry. Their hormones were lying to them.

Dr Eve Van Cauter, who co-authored *Sleep Loss and Obesity*, found that sleep-deprived people consumed an extra 300 calories per day compared to those who slept well. They did not just eat more; they snacked more, driven not only by ghrelin but by a stimulated endocannabinoid system that pushed them towards sugary, high-reward foods. MRI scans showed that after inadequate sleep, the prefrontal cortex, the part of the brain responsible for rational decision-making, went quiet, while the impulsive, emotional brain regions lit up. In other words, sleep deprivation does not just make you hungrier. It makes you worse at resisting the foods you know you should not be eating.

Now layer this on top of the modern food environment we discussed earlier in this book. You are tired. Your hunger hormones are screaming at you. Your rational brain has gone dark. And the entire food industry has been engineered to make you reach for exactly the thing that will spike your insulin the hardest. It is a trap, and poor sleep is the trigger.

Three Nobel Prize-winning scientists, Jeffrey Hall, Michael Rosbash, and Michael Young, were awarded the 2017 Nobel Prize for their work on the circadian clock, the internal timekeeper that governs when your body expects to sleep, wake, eat, and repair. Disrupting this clock, whether through late nights, shift work, or blue light from screens, does not just make you groggy. It throws your cortisol rhythm off, raises your blood pressure, impairs your liver's detoxification cycle, and, yes, drives insulin resistance.

Even your gut microbiome has a circadian rhythm. Certain strains of bacteria fluctuate based on when and what you eat, and a poor diet combined with disrupted sleep can damage these bacterial rhythms, further impairing your metabolic health. Fibre, it turns out, plays a role here too. A fibre-rich diet supports the gut bacteria that help regulate your circadian cycle. Junk food at midnight does the opposite.

I spent decades treating sleep as the enemy of productivity. I championed early mornings and late nights and wore my lack of sleep like a badge of honour. "I'll sleep when I'm dead" was one of my favourite phrases. The research changed my mind completely. A more honest version of that saying would be: "Die sooner because you did not sleep."

Sleep is not a luxury. It is not laziness. It is the foundation your body needs to process glucose, regulate hunger, manage stress, and repair itself at the cellular level. If you are eating well but sleeping badly, you are building a house on sand.

Get your seven hours. Your insulin will thank you.

• • •

The Cortisol Problem

Stress is supposed to save your life. That is what it was designed for. When our ancestors encountered a predator, their bodies triggered a rapid hormonal response: cortisol surged, the liver dumped glucose into the bloodstream, heart rate spiked, muscles tensed, and the body was flooded with fast-burning energy. This is acute stress. It is brief, intense, and purposeful. You either escaped the danger or you did not. Either way, the stress response was over in minutes.

The problem is that modern life has taken a system designed for short bursts and jammed it into the "on" position.

Chronic stress, the kind that comes from money worries, difficult relationships, overwork, loneliness, a toxic boss, or simply the relentless noise of modern living, triggers the same cortisol response. Your liver still dumps glucose. Your blood sugar still rises. But there is no predator to run from. There is no physical exertion to burn through the fuel. The glucose just sits there, and your pancreas has to deal with it. It releases insulin. The insulin forces the sugar into your cells. And if this happens day after day, week after week, year after year, your cells start to resist the signal. Insulin resistance, driven not by food, but by a hormone that was never supposed to be elevated for this long.

The relationship between cortisol and insulin is essentially a tug of war. You can eat perfectly and still develop insulin resistance if your cortisol is chronically elevated. You could follow every piece of dietary advice in this book, eat your fibre first, avoid ultra-processed food, cut back on sugar, and still find that your blood sugar is creeping up, your weight is not shifting, and your energy is flat. If chronic stress is the cause, no amount of broccoli will fix it on its own.

A 2015 study analysed the emotional tone of social media language across different communities and found something remarkable: regions with higher levels of negative, angry, or pessimistic social media posts had higher rates of heart disease mortality than regions with traditional risk factors like smoking or elevated blood pressure. The emotional climate of a community, its collective stress level, was a stronger predictor of cardiovascular death than cigarettes. That is not a metaphor. That is data.

Stress does not just affect your blood sugar. It affects your sleep (which we have just discussed), your appetite (cortisol drives cravings for high-sugar, high-fat foods), your gut health (stress disrupts the microbiome), and your immune function. It is a root cause that quietly feeds every other root cause.

So, what do you do about it?

I am not going to pretend this is simple. Chronic stress is often baked into the structure of someone's life, their job, their finances, their relationships, their caring responsibilities. You cannot always eliminate the source. But you can change how your body responds to it.

Regular physical movement is one of the most effective cortisol regulators there is. Sleep, as we have just covered, keeps cortisol in its natural rhythm. Meditation, yoga, and even deliberate slow breathing have been shown to lower cortisol levels measurably. Building a close circle of people who lift you up rather than drain you makes a genuine difference. So does something as basic as spending time outdoors.

When I travelled to Bhutan, a country that measures Gross National Happiness rather than Gross Domestic Product, I sat with people who lived with almost nothing by Western standards and yet carried an ease about them that most people in the UK would envy. They worried less. They tolerated more. They appreciated impermanence. They laughed more often. They did not chase things they could not control. And their health reflected it.

You do not need to move to the Himalayas. But you do need to take stress seriously as a metabolic threat. It is not something fluffy or optional. It is a hormonal force that drives insulin resistance just as surely as a can of fizzy drink. The difference is that nobody puts a warning label on a stressful job.

If you are doing everything right with your diet and still not seeing results, ask yourself one question: how is my stress? Because cortisol does not care what you had for lunch.

• • •

The Medications Nobody Warned You About

This is the section that will make some people uncomfortable. It made me uncomfortable writing it. But it needs to be said, because millions of people are taking medications that are quietly making their insulin resistance worse, and most of them have never been told.

Let me be absolutely clear before we go any further. I am not a doctor. I am not telling you to stop taking any medication. If your doctor has prescribed something, there is almost certainly a good reason for it. What I am saying is that you deserve to know the full picture, including the side effects that do not always make it into the conversation.

With huge thanks to Dr David Unwin, who helped me collate the research for this section, here is what the science shows.

Statins, the cholesterol-lowering drugs prescribed to millions of people in the UK, have been shown to increase the risk of developing new-onset type 2 diabetes by 10 to 12%. With intensive statin therapy, the risk is even higher. For people already on the borderline of insulin resistance, which, based on everything in this book, is a very large number of adults, statins can be the thing that tips them over the edge. This does not mean statins are always wrong. It means the conversation should be more honest.

Beta-blockers and diuretics, commonly prescribed for blood pressure, can raise fasting blood glucose and HbA1c concentrations. Non-selective beta-blockers and thiazide diuretics show the most significant increases. Again, these drugs serve a purpose. But if you are taking one and your blood sugar is creeping up, it may not be your diet. It may be your prescription.

Antipsychotic drugs, including quetiapine, olanzapine, and clozapine, used for a range of psychiatric conditions, have been shown to increase insulin resistance, promote abdominal fat storage, raise triglycerides, and elevate stress hormones. Clozapine in particular has been linked to the full constellation of insulin resistance: belly fat, high blood pressure, abnormal cholesterol, and elevated blood sugar. Animal studies confirm these drugs significantly disrupt how the body manages glucose, fats, and proteins.

Inhaled corticosteroids, prescribed for asthma and chronic obstructive pulmonary disease (COPD), have been linked to a 34% increase in the risk of developing diabetes. At higher doses, typically used in COPD treatment, the risk climbs further, and these medications have been shown to accelerate the progression of existing diabetes to more severe stages.

Now step back and think about this in the round. We have a population that is already eating too much sugar, too much ultra-processed food, and not enough fibre. Most people are sedentary. Many are stressed and sleep-deprived. And on top of all that, a significant number are taking one or more medications that independently drive insulin resistance. The roots keep multiplying.

What troubles me most is not the medications themselves. Sometimes they are necessary. What troubles me is the lack of joined-up thinking. A patient sees their GP for high blood pressure and gets a beta-blocker. Six months later, their blood sugar is elevated. They go back and get a diabetes diagnosis. Nobody connects the dots. Nobody says, "The drug I gave you for your blood pressure may be contributing to your blood sugar problem." Instead, they get another prescription.

Nina Teicholz put it well: pharmaceutical companies are not profiting if you are getting well. They have no financial interest in your improved health. And while that is not a reason to distrust every drug on the market, it is a reason to ask harder questions and to understand what your medications are actually doing inside your body.

If you are on any of the medications I have listed, please do not panic and please do not stop taking them without speaking to your doctor. But do have the conversation. Ask whether your prescription could be affecting your insulin levels. Ask whether lifestyle changes, the kind outlined in this book and in *The Fibre First Diet*, could reduce your need for the medication over time. Many people who adopt a fibre-first approach, lose weight, and increase their activity levels find that their blood pressure drops, their cholesterol improves, and the case for medication weakens.

That is not a fantasy. Dr David Unwin's NHS practice in Southport has helped hundreds of patients reduce or eliminate their medications through dietary change alone. He was honoured with the NHS Innovator Award for this work. It is possible. But it starts with knowing the full truth about what your pills are doing.

The tree of insulin resistance has many roots. For some people, their medicine cabinet is one of them.

CHAPTER FIFTEEN

What You Can Do Today

• • •

You have read fourteen chapters of science. You have met the tree. You have traced its roots through cancer, Alzheimer's, heart disease, diabetes, fatty liver, infertility, gut disease, and immune dysfunction. You have seen how the government made it worse and how the pharmaceutical industry turned the consequences into a prescription. You have had your eyes opened to how your body actually works, and you have been introduced to the scientists brave enough to say it out loud.

Now it is time to do something about it.

This chapter is deliberately simple. No more biochemistry. No more studies. Just the practical steps you can take, starting today, to begin reversing the damage that insulin resistance has done to your body. Some of these will be familiar from earlier chapters. Some will be new. All of them work.

• • •

Start Here

The One Teaspoon Rule: Before anything else, I want you to hold on to the single most important fact in this entire book. Your bloodstream is designed to carry just one teaspoon of sugar at any time.

Reduce Your Carbohydrates: The most powerful health lever you have is reducing the amount of sugar, grains and starchy carbohydrates in your diet. Not eliminating all carbohydrates. Cauliflower is not the same as a potato. But cutting back on the processed, high-sugar, high-starch foods that spike your insulin.

Start with breakfast. For most people, breakfast is the worst meal of the day. Cereal, toast, orange juice, porridge with honey. It is a blood sugar bomb first thing in the morning. Swap it for eggs, or a protein-based breakfast with no carbohydrates, and you start the day with your insulin low and your body in a position to burn fat rather than store it.

Isabella's KetoSAge study showed that when participants severely reduced carbohydrates, their natural GLP-1 production doubled within weeks. Both hormones improved from the same dietary change. You do not need to go fully ketogenic to benefit, though the deeper you go, the faster the results. Even modest carbohydrate reduction makes a measurable difference.

Eat Fibre First: If you only take one practical lesson from this book, let it be this: change the order in which you eat. Vegetables and fibre first. Then protein. Then carbohydrates last.

When fibre arrives in your gut before carbohydrates, it forms a gel-like barrier that slows the absorption of the sugars that follow. The blood sugar spike is blunted. The insulin response is lower. And the fibre itself stimulates the L-cells in your small intestine to produce GLP-1, your natural appetite hormone. One simple change in the order you eat your food, and you address both hormones at once.

In my Blood Sugar Trial, this single change was enough for more than half the participants to bring their blood sugar and insulin under control without eliminating any food from their diet. They still ate some bread. They still ate some pasta. They just ate their vegetables first.

You can do this at your next meal. It costs nothing. It requires no willpower. And the science behind it is robust.

Discover Glucomannan: If eating fibre first is the foundational principle, glucomannan is the most powerful tool for delivering it. It is a viscous fibre that expands to fifty times its weight in water, forming a thick gel in your stomach that physically stretches the gut wall, triggers your L-cells to produce GLP-1, and slows carbohydrate absorption so your insulin spike is reduced. Both hormones from one fibre.

Glucomannan is the only ingredient that carries approved weight loss claims from the European Food Safety Authority. These are not marketing claims. They are regulatory approvals from one of the most rigorous food safety organisations on earth.

Glucomannan is widely available from health food shops and online. Several brands offer capsules and konjac noodles. Full disclosure: my company Clubwell sells its own range, so take my enthusiasm with a pinch of salt. But the science is independent of the brand, and the EFSA approval applies to the ingredient itself, not any single product.

Avoid Seed Oils: This one surprises most people, because seed oils have been marketed as healthy for decades. Soy oil, sunflower oil, canola oil, safflower oil. These are high in linoleic acid and they are in virtually every processed food you buy. Isabella is clear on this: eliminate them. They drive inflammation, they disrupt your hormonal balance, and they contribute to the metabolic damage that underpins every condition in this book.

What should you use instead? Butter. Olive oil. Coconut oil. Avocado oil. Animal fats. These are the fats your body recognises and can process properly. They are what your grandparents cooked with before the food industry decided that cheap industrial oils were more profitable.

• • •

Go Further

Move After You Eat: A twenty-minute walk after dinner. That is all. You do not need a gym membership. You do not need to run a marathon. Walking creates a gentle one-hertz oscillation in your bones that triggers the production of osteocalcin, a hormone that helps regulate insulin sensitivity. It improves your GLP-1 response after meals. It aids digestion. And it dramatically improves sleep quality, which as we discovered in the last chapter matters more than most people realise.

Hippocrates said it two thousand years ago: walking is man's best medicine. He was not wrong.

If you want to do more, short bursts of resistance exercise are the most effective approach for metabolic health. I am not talking mammoth sessions in a gym. Ten to twenty repetitions of something that challenges each major muscle, then rest. Allow a full day of recovery between sessions. Too much exercise raises cortisol, cortisol raises blood sugar, blood sugar raises insulin, and you end up going backwards.

Fix Your Sleep: We covered the science behind this in the last chapter. Here is what to do about it. The protocol is simple. Phone down one hour before bed. Dark room. Cool temperature. For most people seven to eight hours. Non-negotiable. Get morning sunlight on your face first thing, because it primes your body's circadian clock and sets up the melatonin production you need later that night. Avoid blue light from screens in the evening, because blue light after dark suppresses melatonin, and melatonin is not just a sleep hormone. It is one of the most powerful antioxidants your body produces, protecting your mitochondria overnight.

Sleep is not a luxury. It is metabolic infrastructure. Treat it accordingly.

Manage Your Stress: You might eat perfectly and sleep well and still carry stubborn weight if your cortisol is chronically elevated. Cortisol tells your liver to release glucose. Glucose triggers insulin. And if that cycle runs all day, every day, it does not matter how clean your plate is.

You cannot always remove the source of stress. But you can change how your body processes it. A daily walk helps. So does deliberate slow breathing, even five minutes of it. Build a circle of people who lift you rather than drain you. Spend time outdoors. And if you find yourself grinding through each week fuelled by caffeine and anxiety, take that as seriously as you would a bad blood test result. Stress is not a feeling. It is a hormonal event, and it drives insulin resistance through exactly the same pathway as sugar.

Watch the Right Numbers: If you go to your GP and ask them to check your metabolic health, they will almost certainly look at your HbA1c for blood sugar and your liver enzymes. But as we discussed in Chapter 10, the reference ranges that define normal are dangerously lenient.

If you can get hold of a continuous glucose monitor, even for two or three weeks, the education is extraordinary. Seeing in real time what a bowl of cereal does to your blood sugar versus what eggs and vegetables do is worth more than a hundred books. It makes the abstract science in these pages viscerally, personally real.

But blood sugar, as important as it is, is only one piece of the picture. Doctors and researchers around the world now recognise a cluster of five measurements that together define something called metabolic syndrome. These are the five numbers that tell you whether insulin resistance has already taken hold in your body. They are not exotic or expensive. Most of them can be tested by your GP with a routine blood test, and there are plenty of devices available that allow you to measure these from home. If any three of the five are outside the healthy range, you have metabolic syndrome. And if you have metabolic syndrome, you have insulin resistance, which means the tree we have been talking about throughout this book is already growing inside you.

Five Numbers That Tell You Everything: Let me walk you through each one, because understanding why these five measurements matter is the difference between hoping you are healthy and knowing where you currently are.

Waist-to-height ratio. Forget BMI. A bodybuilder and a couch potato can have the same BMI, which tells you everything you need to know about how useful it is. Your waist-to-height ratio is far more revealing, because it measures visceral fat, the fat that wraps around your organs and drives insulin resistance. The measurement is simple: take a piece of string, cut it to your height, fold it in half, and wrap it around your waist. If it does not meet comfortably, your visceral fat is too high. As a number, you want your waist circumference to be less than half your height. A six-foot man should have a waist under 36 inches. A five-foot-five woman should be under 32.5 inches. This single measurement correlates more strongly with metabolic disease than almost anything your GP will test.

Blood pressure. You already know high blood pressure is dangerous. What most people do not realise is that insulin resistance is one of its primary drivers. When insulin is chronically elevated, it causes your kidneys to retain sodium, which increases fluid volume and pushes your blood pressure up. It also stiffens your arterial walls over time. So, when your blood pressure is elevated, it is not just a heart risk. It is a metabolic warning. Ideally you want to see something around 120 over 80, though what matters most is the trend over time.

Fasting blood glucose. This is the amount of sugar in your blood after an overnight fast, before you have eaten anything. It is the simplest and most direct measure of how well your body is managing that one teaspoon limit we talked about earlier. A healthy fasting glucose is below 5.0 mmol/L. Between 5.5 and 6.9 is pre-diabetic. Above 7.0 is diabetic. But here is the important thing: by the time fasting glucose is elevated, insulin resistance has usually been building for years. That is why it works best alongside the other four markers rather than on its own.

Triglycerides. Triglycerides are the fat molecules circulating in your blood. When you eat more sugar or refined carbohydrates than your body can burn, your liver converts the excess into triglycerides. High triglycerides are a direct signal that your liver is overwhelmed and your insulin is working overtime. You want your level below 1.7 mmol/L. Above 2.3 and you are in territory where your body is clearly struggling to process what you are eating.

HDL cholesterol. This is the one cholesterol number that genuinely matters for metabolic health. HDL particles help clear excess cholesterol from your arteries and transport it back to the liver. When HDL is high, it is a sign your metabolism is functioning well. When it is low, it almost always tracks with insulin resistance. You want your HDL above 1.0 mmol/L for men and above 1.3 mmol/L for women, as levels lower than this are associated with higher cardiovascular risk.

There is also a powerful shortcut that many doctors still underuse: the triglyceride to HDL ratio. Take your fasting triglycerides and divide them by your HDL (both in mmol/L). A ratio below about 1.5 is typically seen in people with very good metabolic health, whereas a ratio above 3.0 is strongly associated with insulin resistance and other metabolic problems in many studies. It is one of the most useful proxy markers we have for insulin sensitivity, but it should be interpreted alongside other blood tests and clinical context rather than as a diagnosis on its own.

Together, these five markers paint a picture that no single blood test can. A CGM shows you what sugar is doing right now. These combined tell you what sugar has been doing to your body over months and years. That is the difference between a snapshot and a forecast.

And here is the good news. Every single one of these numbers can change. This is not a life sentence. It is a snapshot of where you are right now, today, based on what you have been eating and how you have been living. Your waist measurement, your blood pressure, your fasting glucose, your triglycerides, your HDL. None of them are fixed. They are all responding to what you put on your plate. People who switch to fibre-first eating or move more towards a ketogenic lifestyle, routinely see their triglycerides drop, their HDL rise, their blood pressure normalise, and their waist shrink, often within weeks. So do not look at these numbers and think, "I do not want to know." Look at them and think, "Now I know where I am starting from." Because there is something far worse than a bad score: it's a bad score you never checked.

• • •

Go All In

Consider a Ketogenic Lifestyle: If you are ready to go the whole way, a well-formulated ketogenic diet is the most powerful tool any of us have found. Isabella, Ben and I are all passionate about it, and the reason is simple: if you are in ketosis, it is proof that your insulin is low. You do not have to guess. You do not have to hope. You can measure it with a keto monitor, whether that is a breath monitor, a blood finger-prick device, or a simple urine strip. If the reading says you are in ketosis, your insulin is down and your body is burning its own fat for fuel.

And if you do go fully ketogenic, it is only fair for me to say that you do not have to worry about counting your fibre. Fibre is the antidote to sugar. If you have removed the sugar, the fibre becomes optional.

Tell Someone: This might seem like an odd inclusion in a chapter about practical health steps, but it might be the most important one of all. Tell someone what you have learned. A partner, a friend, a parent, a colleague. Not to lecture them. Just to share it.

Every person who reads this book and changes has gained something: understanding. But every person who reads this book and tells one other person has started something bigger. Because the system I described in the previous chapters, the dietary guidelines, the pharmaceutical machine, the processed food industry, that system depends on ignorance. It depends on people not knowing that their blood should carry just one teaspoon of sugar.

The moment people know, the system loses its power. And the moment enough people know, the system has to change.

• • •

The Final Evidence

There are thousands of studies I could point you to, but if I had to choose just one, it would be a Swedish population study published in the journal GeroScience in 2023.

Sweden keeps some of the most meticulous health records in the world, tracking its citizens across decades. That makes it an ideal country for this kind of research. The question the researchers set out to answer was simple: what do the longest-lived people have in common?

They were not looking at lifestyle choices or diet diaries or exercise habits. They were looking at blood. Specifically, they wanted to know which biomarkers most consistently showed up in people who survived beyond 100.

Three variables stood out above all others.

The first was good glucose control. The longest-lived people kept their blood sugar levels low and stable throughout their lives. This should not surprise anyone who has read this far into this book. If you control your glucose, you control your insulin. If you control your insulin, you protect every organ in your body from the cascade of damage we have been describing chapter after chapter.

The second finding was low uric acid. High uric acid is increasingly being linked to metabolic syndrome, gout, kidney disease, and cardiovascular problems. It rises when the body is overloaded with fructose and alcohol, both of which are processed by the liver in ways that drive insulin resistance. Low uric acid, in other words, is another marker of a metabolically healthy body.

The third finding is the one that will raise eyebrows. The longest-lived people had high total cholesterol.

Let that sink in for a moment. We live in a world where the moment your cholesterol creeps above a certain number, you are handed a prescription for a statin. Millions of people take cholesterol-lowering medication every single day. And yet, when researchers looked at the blood of the people who actually lived the longest, they found higher cholesterol, not lower.

This is not as contradictory as it sounds. Cholesterol is not a toxin. It is a molecule of life. Every cell membrane in your body is built from it. Every sex hormone, testosterone, oestrogen, progesterone, is constructed from cholesterol. Your mitochondria, the energy factories inside every cell, need cholesterol to function. Your immune system uses LDL cholesterol to fight infections. When you lower cholesterol aggressively through medication, you are not just lowering a number on a blood test. You are potentially compromising the very structures that keep your body running.

None of this means cholesterol cannot become a problem. But it does mean that the blanket war on cholesterol, the idea that lower is always better, may be one of the most damaging oversimplifications in modern medicine. The Swedish data suggests that what matters most is not whether your cholesterol is high or low, but whether your metabolism is working properly. And the single best indicator of that? Glucose control. Which brings us right back to insulin.

So why is the entire medical establishment still so fixated on LDL cholesterol? I think you have to follow the money. You can create a drug that lowers cholesterol. Statins are one of the most profitable medications in the history of pharmaceuticals. There is a huge amount of money to be made in prescribing a pill that brings a number down on a blood test. But there is no money to be made in telling people to lower their blood sugar through food. In fact, quite the opposite. If people stopped eating the processed carbohydrates that spike their insulin, entire industries would collapse. The food companies that sell the products that make us sick. The pharmaceutical companies that sell the drugs that manage the symptoms. Nobody in that chain has any financial interest in you simply eating better.

The longest-lived people in Sweden were simply metabolically healthy. Their insulin was doing its job properly. Their glucose stayed stable. Their bodies were not inflamed. And their cholesterol was left alone to do what it is supposed to do: build, repair, and protect.

If you want to live longer, the evidence from Sweden says the same thing this entire book has been saying. Fix your insulin. Everything else follows.

• • •

A Final Word

I started writing this book because my parents developed type 2 diabetes. My mum went on to develop Alzheimer's. My dad lived for years with gout, erectile dysfunction, and high blood pressure before anyone thought about type 2 diabetes. By the time they were diagnosed, the damage had been accumulating for decades.

I wrote it because for 30 years I was obese and I spent years believing it was my fault. That I just needed to eat less and move more. It was not until I understood insulin, and GLP-1, and the tree that connects them to virtually every chronic disease, that everything changed. And once it changed for me, I could not keep it to myself.

Isabella Cooper and Ben Bikman gave me the science. The KetoSAge study, the Fibre First research, the House of Lords paper, the interviews that became the backbone of this book. They are two of the bravest, most rigorous scientists I have ever met, and without them, this book would not exist. I am not a doctor. I am a businessman who became obsessed with a problem and refused to accept the answers I was being given.

But the science is clear. Insulin resistance is the trunk. The branches of modern disease grow from it. And the tree can be cut down, not with drugs, not with injections, but with food, movement, sleep, and knowledge.

It was always the insulin.

CHAPTER SIXTEEN

Where to Go from Here

• • •

If this book has opened your eyes, the best thing you can do now is keep them open. The people and organisations below are the ones I trust most to help you do that.

Dr Isabella Cooper

Isabella's research is the backbone of this book, and there is plenty more where it came from. Her landmark KetoSAge study, which examined what happens when long-term ketosis is suppressed in healthy women, has produced a series of published papers that are free to read online. If you want to go deeper into the science of insulin resistance, hyperinsulinaemia, and how they connect to ageing and chronic disease, her work is the place to start.

Her key published papers include:

- "Ketosis Suppression and Ageing (KetoSAge): The Effects of Suppressing Ketosis in Long Term Keto-Adapted Non-Athletic Females"

- "Ketosis Suppression and Ageing (KetoSAge) Part 2: The Effect of Suppressing Ketosis on Biomarkers Associated with Ageing, HOMA-IR, Leptin, Osteocalcin"

- "Rethinking Fragility Fractures in Type 2 Diabetes: The Link Between Hyperinsulinaemia and Osteofragilitas"

- "Metabolic Phenotypes and Step by Step Evolution of Type 2 Diabetes: A New Paradigm"

- "Bio-Hacking Better Health: Leveraging Metabolic Biochemistry to Maximise Healthspan"

You can find all of her published research by searching "Isabella Cooper" on Google Scholar (scholar.google.com) or PubMed (pubmed.ncbi.nlm.nih.gov). Many of her papers are published in open-access journals, which means you can read them for free.

• • •

Professor Ben Bikman

If you have not already read Ben's book *Why We Get Sick*, do yourself a favour and order it today. It is one of those rare books that takes complex metabolic science and makes it not just understandable but genuinely compelling. Every home should have a copy.

Beyond the book, Ben is generous with his time and knowledge online. His YouTube channel is packed with interviews, lectures, and explanations that will deepen everything you have read in these pages. Search for "Ben Bikman" on YouTube and you will find hundreds of hours of free education on insulin resistance, ketosis, metabolic flexibility, and why the conventional dietary advice has been getting it so wrong for so long.

• • •

Watch Our Conversations

You can also watch my in-depth interviews with both Isabella and Ben on the Clubwell YouTube channel. These are the conversations that shaped much of this book, and hearing Isabella and Ben explain these concepts in their own words brings a different dimension to what you have read on these pages. Search for "Clubwell" on YouTube or visit youtube.com/@Clubwell to find them.

• • •

The Public Health Collaboration (PHC)

The PHC is a UK charity that exists to do something remarkably simple: get the truth about nutrition and health into public policy. We challenge outdated dietary guidelines, promote evidence-based health advice, and campaign for real change in how the nation approaches food and metabolic disease. If you believe, as I do, that the current system is failing millions of people, then the PHC is fighting in your corner.

You can support our work by becoming a member. Visit phcuk.org to find out more. Even if you simply follow what we do, it will keep you informed and connected to a community that cares about the same things you have just read about.

Acknowledgements

Writing this book would not have been possible without a constellation of remarkable individuals, beyond the superstars that are Isabella Cooper and Ben Bikman, all united by a shared passion for enhancing global wellbeing. The creation of this book and the evolution of my own health owe immense gratitude to these guiding stars.

Dr David Unwin, you are a trailblazer in enhancing our understanding of type 2 diabetes, and your innovative sugar charts have been an invaluable resource. Your significant role at the Public Health Collaboration alongside Director Sam Feltham is nothing short of transformative. Sam, your dedication to reshaping our nation's health is commendable.

Dr Ben Bocchicchio, your myth-busting on exercise and diet, especially around BMI, has been enlightening. Patrick McKeown, Dr Anna Symonds, Dr Nicole Avena, Dr Peter Brukner, Patrick Holford, Dr Mark Cucuzzella, Dr James DiNicolantonio, Dr Deborah Colson, Dr Dominic D'Agostino, Dr Robert Lustig, Dr James Goolnik, nutritionist Hannah Richards, Dr Jason Fung, Dr Mary Newport, Professor Tim Noakes, and Dr Malcolm Kendrick: your collective wisdom has been a guiding light.

To the late Dr Michael Mosley, whose work in opening the world's eyes to intermittent fasting was groundbreaking. Emma Porter, your culinary talents and countless hours of collaboration have been invaluable. To the Caldesi family, our discussions on low-carb cooking have been both delicious and enlightening.

Tom Watson, your journey and insights into the intersection of health and politics have been invaluable. To the trio of investigative journalists Gary Taubes, Nina Teicholz, and Jerome Burne, your time and contributions to my podcast were invaluable, and along with Dr David Diamond and Dr Eric Berg, your dedication in uncovering the tricks, deceit, and campaigns used by the food and pharmaceutical industry will never be forgotten. Dr Steve Witherly, thank you for illuminating the food industry's tactics. Patrick Holden CBE, your insights into soil health and sustainable farming have been eye-opening.

Dr Ian Lake and Jon Furniss, your organisation of our fasting experiments and education on type 1 diabetes have been transformative. A special thanks to Dr Ali Ibrahim for joining me on countless miles of cycling and walking adventures. Our endless discussions about the deceptive food industry, the complexities of eating disorders, and your remarkable collaboration with Dr Agnes Ayton on researching the Western diet have been invaluable and deeply appreciated.

Dr Jen Unwin, Dr Nicole Avena, and Dr Vera Tarman, your work on food addiction has been revolutionary and will certainly help shape food education for the future. Dr Dan Maggs and Dr Shan Hussain, your endless hours of sharing knowledge are deeply appreciated.

A special thanks to Dr Shawn Baker for your valuable participation in my panel at the PHC conference. Your presence and contributions significantly enriched the event, especially the debate we held with you and Dr Anthony Chaffee on the merits of the carnivore diet. My sincere appreciation for speaking at our conference also goes to Dr Georgia Ede, Dr David Cavan, Dr Zsofia Clemens, Professor Roy Taylor, and Dr Bob Gill for their invaluable contributions.

To my blood sugar trial research team: Nick Davies, Barry Wiggins, Kim Heighway and her daughter Olivia, Laura Palmer, Brooke Foster-Roantree, Liam Coakes, David Reid, Joshua Morris, and Jake Thompson. Your support and willingness to consume such a diversity of food on our many trials is truly appreciated.

Dr Boz, your story of reversing your mother's cancer and our conversations have been motivating.

To my beloved seven children, this book is a testament to my hope for your healthy lives. My wife, for her unwavering support. My parents, whose strength in the face of illness drives my commitment to this message. To my grandchildren, may the wisdom in these pages guide you. And to my late grandmother and Auntie Avis, tragically swept away by cancer in their fifties, you remain in my heart always.

To those whose names have not been individually etched in these pages, please know your influence resonates in every word. This book is a mosaic of contributions from each of you, a testament to our collective mission to reshape health and consciousness. Thank you, from the depths of my heart, for being the architects of this book.

www.ingramcontent.com/pod-product-compliance
Lightning Source LLC
La Vergne TN
LVHW100303210926
848480LV00003B/1005
9781918852004